Lecture Notes on Haematology

Lecture Notes on Haematology

N. C. HUGHES-JONES
D.M. Ph.D. M.A. M.R.C.P.

Member of the Scientific Staff,
Medical Research Council's
Mechanism in Tumour Immunity Unit,
Hon. Consultant Haematologist,
Department of Haematology,
Addenbrooke's Hospital,
Hon. Lecturer, Department of Pathology,
Cambridge

FOURTH EDITION

BLACKWELL SCIENTIFIC PUBLICATIONS

OXFORD LONDON EDINBURGH
BOSTON PALO ALTO MELBOURNE

Editorial Offices:
Osney Mead, Oxford OX2 0EL
8 John Street, London WC1N 2ES
9 Forrest Road, Edinburgh EH1 2QH
52 Beacon Street, Boston
Massachusetts 02108, U.S.A.
706 Cowper Street, Palo Alto
California 94301, U.S.A.
99 Barry Street, Carlton
Victoria 3053, Australia

First published 1970
Second edition 1973
Reprinted 1975
Third edition 1979
Reprinted 1980
Fourth edition 1984

Set by Preface Ltd
Salisbury, Wiltshire
Printed and bound by
Billing & Sons Ltd, Worcester

DISTRIBUTORS

U.S.A.
Blackwell Mosby Book Distributors
11830 Westline Industrial Drive
St Louis, Missouri 63141

Canada
Blackwell Mosby Book Distributors
120 Melford Drive, Scarborough
Ontario M1B 2X4

Australia
Blackwell Scientific Book
Distributors
31 Advantage Road, Highett
Victoria 3190

British Library
Cataloguing in Publication Data
Hughes-Jones, Nevin Campbell
Lecture notes on haematology.
4th ed.
1. Blood—Diseases
I. Title
616.1′5 RC636

ISBN 0-632-01302-8

Contents

Preface to Fourth Edition

All chapters have been revised in this edition to include the relevant advances that have appeared in the last few years. The most significant of these is in our understanding of the thalassaemias and these have been included in the chapter on haemolytic anaemias. As I have said in a previous preface, the aim of the book is, first, to provide sufficient information so that, on qualification, the common haematological diseases can be diagnosed and treated without outside help; secondly, to make known the general principles of the uncommon diseases so that further practical knowledge can be acquired and acted upon.

The text was originally written for undergraduates as at that time (1970) only advanced text-books on haematology were available. Since then, it has become apparent that it is also of value to those who are taking higher examinations in other subjects and require a background of basic haematology.

I am extremely grateful to Dr Barbara Bain for her very thorough reading of the text, for pointing out errors and for making amendments and suggestions to improve clarity, and also to Professor Sunita Wickramasinghe for his comments on the chapter on leukaemia. I would also like to thank Mrs Joan Payne for so patiently typing (and retyping) the manuscript.

Cambridge,
March 1984

N. C. Hughes-Jones

Preface to First Edition

These lecture notes are designed to supply the basic knowledge of both the clinical and laboratory aspects of haematological diseases and blood transfusion. The content is broadly similar to that of the course given to medical students by the Department of Haematology at St Mary's Hospital Medical School. References have been cited so that those who require to extend their knowledge in any particular field can do so. Most of the journals and books that are mentioned are those commonly found in every library.

At the end of each chapter I have supplied a list of objectives in studying each disease. There are two main purposes in these objectives. First, they facilitate the learning process, since the process of acquisition, retention and recall of data is greatly helped if the facts and concepts are centred around a particular objective. Secondly, many objectives are closely related to the practical problems encountered in the diagnosis and treatment of patients. For instance, the following objects: 'to understand the method of differentiation of megaloblastic anaemia due to vitamin B_{12} deficiency from that due to folate deficiency' and 'to understand the basis for the differentiation of leukaemia into acute and chronic forms based on the clinical picture and on the peripheral blood findings' are practical problems encountered frequently in the haematology laboratory. A point of more immediate interest to the undergraduate is that examiners setting either multiple choice or essay questions will be searching for the same knowledge that is required in answering the objectives.

I should like to thank Professor P. L. Mollison, Dr P. Barkhan, Dr I. Chanarin, Dr G. J. Jenkins and Dr M. S. Rose for their criticism and helpful suggestions during the preparation of the manuscript and Mrs Inge Barnett for typing the several drafts and final typescript.

St Mary's Hospital Medical School,   N. C. Hughes-Jones
January 1970

Chapter 1
Iron Metabolism and Iron Deficiency Anaemia

Physiology of iron

Distribution of iron in the body

Iron is an essential component of haemoglobin and of the respiratory enzymes and is thus present in all cells. Deficiency of iron results in inadequate haemoglobin production and consequent impairment of red cell formation. Most of the signs and symptoms of iron deficiency are due to anaemia. It has been suggested that the feeling of tiredness and general malaise that may accompany severe iron deficiency is the result of a fall in the concentration of iron-containing respiratory enzymes (Beutler *et al*. 1960). The deleterious effects of mild iron-deficiency anaemia has been demonstrated in rubber plantation workers in Java, who were paid on piece rates. Work output correlated with haemoglobin concentration, and treatment with iron raised both haemoglobin values and the amount of work achieved (Viteri & Torun 1974).

About two-thirds of the iron in the body is found in the red cells: 1 ml of red cells contains approximately 1 mg of iron, so that an adult has about 2 g of iron in the red cell mass. About 0·15 g are present as myoglobin and respiratory enzymes. The stores of iron are found in macrophages of the spleen and bone marrow and in both Kupffer and parenchymal cells of the liver. The stores of iron vary from 0 to 1 g or more. Iron is always found in the body bound to a protein. This is a protective device, since ionized iron is toxic. Storage iron is only found within cells and is in the two forms, ferritin and haemosiderin. Ferritin is composed of a protein shell and encloses an iron core containing up to 4000 molecules of iron. Haemosiderin is composed of degraded ferritin which has partly lost its protein shell and the molecules have aggregated. Ferritin is water soluble and is thus not seen on ordinary histological sections as it is removed during the preparations of the slide. Haemosiderin on the other hand can be seen as golden-brown granules in unstained preparations or as blue granules inside reticulum cells

1

when stained with ferricyanide (Prussian Blue reaction). The two forms of iron both increase or decrease together with changes in the total body stores.

Dynamic state of body iron

Iron is continuously circulating through the plasma bound to the protein, transferrin, and the major part of this iron is derived from the daily destruction of approximately 20 ml of red cells, which liberates 20 mg of iron. There is also a further 10–15 mg of iron carried through the plasma daily. This iron is derived from stores and tissues. Iron which is released into the plasma is rapidly removed by haemopoietic tissue in the bone marrow but part goes to stores and to new tissue formation. The half-time for passage of iron through the circulation is approximately 100 min, so that only about 3 mg are in the plasma at any given time.

Iron absorption

An average diet contains approximately 10–20 mg of iron per day, mostly in organic form but there is some in inorganic form. Iron is widely distributed and is present in both vegetables and meat, the concentration being higher in the latter. Adults who have normal iron stores absorb approximately 5–10% of their total intake, i.e. 0·5–2 mg/day. The precise amount absorbed is dependent on the chemical form of iron in the food. Iron in the form of haem is absorbed best as the haem molecule is taken up by intestinal cells, and only after absorption is the iron split from the porphyrin ring. Non-haem iron is less well absorbed as it can be readily bound by inhibiting ligands, such as phytates. Ferric iron is reduced to the ferrous form before absorption; hence oral iron is given therapeutically as the ferrous salt. Ascorbic acid is an excellent promotor of absorption of non-haem iron, partly because it is a reducing agent and partly because it forms a small molecular complex with it, which aids adsorption. Iron is absorbed in the upper half of the small intestine, a point to remember when there is surgical removal in this area.

It has long been established that the incidence of gastric atrophy and of achlorhydria is higher in patients with iron-deficiency anaemia than in normal people, but there has been a great deal of argument as to the relationship between the gastric changes and the iron deficiency. There are in fact two questions to be answered. First, does gastric atrophy lead to iron deficiency or does iron deficiency cause the gastric atrophy? Secondly, if the gastric atrophy is an aetiological factor, is it the achlorhydria which is responsible for the failure to absorb iron or is it the absence of some other factor? There are two pieces of evidence that are pertinent to these questions.

1 In most instances the gastric atrophy is irreversible and there is no return to normality after cure of the iron deficiency. This indicates that the gastric atrophy is the primary factor.

2 It is reasonably well-established that inorganic iron is less well absorbed in iron-deficient patients with achlorhydria than in those who secrete HCl. Thus, Goldberg *et al.* (1963) found that only 18% of a tracer dose of $^{59}FeCl_3$ was absorbed in iron-deficient patients with histamine-fast achlorhydria compared to 57% absorbed in those with normal gastric secretion. The evidence suggests that where iron-deficiency anaemia is accompanied by achlorhydria and gastric atrophy, the gastric lesion may well be the aetiological factor leading to iron deficiency. The presence of HCl does appear to play a role in promoting iron absorption, and no convincing evidence for any other factor in the gastric secretion has been found.

Absorption of iron does not remain constant at 5–10% of total intake but is altered according to both the state of iron stores and to the rate of haemopoiesis. When iron intake is in excess of that required for growth, gestation and losses, the iron stores are laid down in the liver, spleen and bone marrow. As iron stores increase, the rate of accumulation decreases, partly due to a slowing in the rate of absorption and partly due to increased loss as the result of an increase in iron content of cells shed from the body. Eventually an equilibrium is reached when iron stores remain constant. The upper limit of normal iron stores in healthy people is about 1 g. On the other hand, when iron stores are depleted, the absorptive mechanism is stimulated and the percentage of iron absorbed is increased so that, in iron deficiency, absorption may rise to over 50% of total intake.

Iron is absorbed from the gut contents into the epithelial cells where it is either passed on to the plasma transferrin or remains within the cells and combines with apoferritin to form ferritin. The transfer of iron from the epithelial cells into the plasma is controlled by an unidentified mechanism which responds to iron requirements, the rate being rapid when stores are reduced. Iron present as ferritin which is not required by the body remains in the epithelial cells until desquamation takes place and the iron is then excreted in the faeces: see Bothwell (1968) for a short review of iron absorption, and Aisen (1982).

Iron loss

There is no specific excretory mechanism for iron. Nevertheless, there is an inevitable daily loss of iron as a result of the continuous exfoliation of gut and skin epithelial cells, all of which have iron-containing enzymes. In adults, this loss is approximately 0·6 mg/day (Finch & Loden 1959). The extra loss in women due to menstruation and pregnancy is discussed later (p. 7).

Iron-depletion and iron-deficiency anaemia

As body iron stores are depleted, two phases can be recognized. The first stage is *iron depletion without anaemia*, when stores are exhausted but the haemoglobin concentration is either unaffected or has only fallen slightly so that, although it is slightly below the normal for that individual, it is still within the generally accepted normal range as defined by WHO criteria (see p. 157). Further depletion of body iron results in an insufficient amount of iron being present to maintain the red cell mass, haemoglobin concentration then falls below the normal range and *iron deficiency anaemia* results.

In any given population, there are approximately equal numbers of people with iron depletion alone and with iron-deficiency anaemia. It is probable that the course of events in the development of iron depletion without anaemia is as follows. An individual woman with iron stores may be in iron equilibrium by absorbing 10% of the iron in her diet. Should she then go into negative iron balance as a result of chronic haemorrhage, iron stores will diminish and when they are finally depleted, iron absorption will be stimulated and rise to a value which now brings her back into iron balance, but insufficient to accumulate iron stores. This state would then be maintained until the equilibrium was altered again. For instance, if the rate of iron loss increased still further so that it exceeded the rate at which it could be absorbed from the diet, then anaemia would ensue. On the other hand, if iron loss decreased, then iron would start to accumulate again, but this would lead to reduced absorption and a new equilibrium would be reached.

Iron-deficiency anaemia is also referred to by the descriptive term of hypochromic anaemia because the red cells have a reduced haemoglobin content, but this term is imprecise as it includes anaemias of different aetiology, notably thalassaemia and the anaemia associated with chronic infection and malignancies.

Iron-deficiency anaemia appears most frequently during two periods of life; namely, in infants of both sexes and in women during the child-bearing period.

Iron-deficiency in infancy
Iron deficiency is frequently found between the ages of 6 months and 5 years, the highest incidence being found at about 12 months. Davis *et al.* (1960) found that about half of a group of West Indian infants and one-quarter of European infants living in London had iron deficiency, as judged by the finding of a mean cell haemoglobin concentration (MCHC) of below 30 g/dl. After the age of 3 years, iron deficiency is less common but not insignificant. Among people of modest income in the U.S., approximately 5% of the children aged 5–11 years had iron deficiency anaemia and a further 10% had iron depletion without anaemia (Cook *et al.* 1976).

There are two factors which predispose to iron deficiency in infancy; namely, inadequate iron stores at birth and inadequate amount of iron in the diet. Approximately half the iron stores are deposited in the last month of fetal life, and thus prematurity due to any cause means that body iron stores may become depleted before the child starts on iron-rich solid food. The growing child during the first year has been estimated to need 0·5–0·9 mg of iron each day (Burman 1982); this cannot be supplied by either human or cow's milk, since both sources have low concentrations of iron and 5–9 pints would be required to provide sufficient iron for the child's daily needs.

A 4-kg child is provided with sufficient iron stores to last for 6 months. It is thus important that the child should be started on iron-rich foods by this time. On the other hand, a 2·5-kg baby has only sufficient iron to grow to 4 or 5 kg, which occurs before solid food is given and hence liquid iron supplements must be supplied.

Inadequate iron intake may continue once solid food has been started. It is for this reason that specially prepared infant foods, such as those based on cereals, have an artificially raised iron content. It is thought that about 10 mg of iron per day is required during the first 2 years of life; a substantial proportion of infants in this age group in the English population receives less than 10 mg of iron in their daily diet at the present time.

Iron deficiency in adolescents and adults

Prevalence
The incidence of iron deficiency has always been found to be much higher in women than in men, especially during the fertile years. Thus, Jacobs *et al.* (1969) investigated a random sample of adult women in Wales and found that 12% of the women had iron depletion alone and 10% of the women also had iron deficiency anaemia. In a study in both Latin America and in the North Western U.S.A., approximately 10% of women were iron depleted and a further 10% were also anaemic (Cook *et al.* 1971; Cook *et al.* 1976).

The incidence of iron defiency in males is much lower. In a sample from Wales, 4·5% had iron depletion and 1·5% were also anaemic (Jacobs *et al.* 1969). Brumfitt (1960) found an incidence of approximately 1% in 17–21-year-old male recruits for the Royal Army Medical Corps. Elwood *et al.* (1964b) found the prevalence of iron deficiency anaemia for 14-year-old school children in Cardiff to be 2·4% for boys and 4·2% for the girls.

Fry (1961) investigated the incidence of iron-deficiency anaemia in general practice and found that most males present with iron deficiency before the age of 10, or after 50 years. In distinction to this, the peak period of presentation in women is during and immediately after the child-bearing period, the peak period being 30–50 years.

Giles & Burton (1960) found that 66% of pregnant women had haemoglobin concentrations below 11·8 g/dl when first seen in the antenatal clinic. Based on the response to iron therapy it was concluded that the majority of these women were iron deficient, although folic acid deficiency and haemodilution were also aetiological factors in the anaemia.

Causes of iron deficiency
Absence of iron stores results when the rate of absorption of iron is insufficient to replace iron lost from the body. Inadequate absorption may be due to a low iron content in the diet or to

impairment of intestinal absorptive mechanisms. On the other hand, loss of iron through haemorrhage may occur at a greater rate than replacement from a normal diet by a normal absorptive mechanism.

Since the incidence of iron deficiency is so much higher in women than in males, it is reasonable to assign the cause to excessive loss of iron through menstruation and child birth, and this assumption is supported by the evidence which is available at the present time. Three reports may be cited. First, that of Scott & Pritchard (1967) who investigated 114 college women aged 19–25 years in Texas. One-quarter of the women had no demonstrable iron stores in the marrow, about two-thirds of the women had iron stores of less than 350 mg, and only 5% had sufficient stainable marrow iron to suggest that the stores were in the range of 500–1000 mg, which is the generally accepted level for normal iron stores.

Secondly, the measurement of blood loss during menstruation shows that the rate of loss in many women is sufficient to reduce the iron stores rapidly. Halberg et al. (1966) studied women working in a factory and found the mean loss of blood was 34 ml (range 2–200 ml) with each period. He considered that this might underestimate the loss in the population as a whole, which may be as high as an average of 43 ml in each period. The group of women losing more than 60 ml with each period showed a reduction in haemoglobin concentration and MCHC, a fall in plasma iron concentration and a rise in total iron binding capacity compared to those losing smaller amounts. These findings suggest that many women losing 60 ml or more are depleted of iron stores (Fig. 1.1). Ten of the 137 women had iron-deficiency anaemia (haemoglobin concentration less than 12 g/dl) and the average menstrual loss of these iron-deficient women, 58 ml, was considerably higher than the mean for the group as a whole. The diagram shown in Fig. 1.2 taken from Jacobs et al. (1965) shows the monthly menstrual loss and the iron requirements in 151 normal women. The daily iron requirements are based on a value of 10% iron absorption from the diet, and it can be seen that women losing 80 ml of blood or more require 21 mg of iron or over as a daily intake, i.e. more than is present in a normal diet.

Thirdly, there is the evidence of Chanarin & Rothman (1965) who examined 49 marrow biopsies from women towards the end of pregnancy, including 16 women who had normal haemotologial

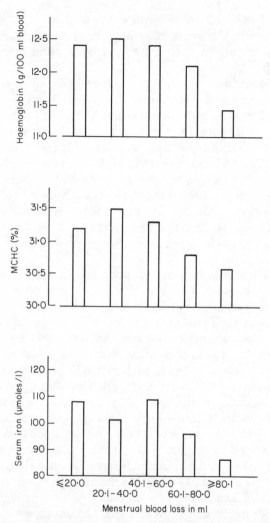

Fig. 1.1. Mean values of haemoglobin concentration, MCHC and serum iron concentration in relation to menstrual blood loss. Redrawn from Halberg *et al.* (1966).

values. Only 4 of the patients had demonstrable iron stores, and all of these were on iron supplements during pregnancy.

The total amount of iron required by the mother during each pregnancy is high, being of the order of 500–700 mg. The fetus requires approximately 250 mg and the rest is lost in the placenta and through haemorrhage. Thus, women during the child-bearing

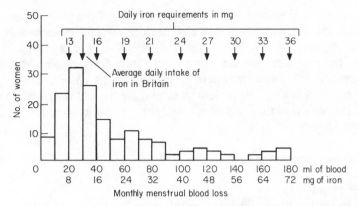

Fig. 1.2. Menstrual blood loss in 151 normal women. The daily iron requirements are calculated on the basis that 10% of the iron in the diet is absorbed. Adapted from Jacobs *et al.* (1965).

period require to absorb each day about 2–3 mg more than men, in whom the basic requirement is about 0·6 mg/day. This is more than can be absorbed from a normal unsupplemented diet and unless the mother starts pregnancy with more than about 200 mg, iron depletion will almost certainly occur. As a group, women of child-bearing age will thus have lower iron stores than men of a similar age, and it is probably only those women who have a high iron intake and small menstrual losses who are able to maintain adequate iron stores.

Of the causes of iron deficiency other than menstruation (or abnormal uterine bleeding) and child-birth, an inadequate diet and diseases of the gastrointestinal tract predominate. In a retrospective review of 378 patients with iron deficiency by Beveridge *et al.* (1965), 19% were found to be due to a poor diet. Gastrointestinal bleeding due to various causes accounted for about 40% and gastrectomy and steatorrhoea accounted for a further 14% of cases.

Gastrectomy is frequently followed by iron deficiency: Tovey & Clark (1980) found 40% of patients were anaemic 9–14 years after a gastrectomy and that 53% relapsed after one course of iron therapy. Iron deficiency in these patients is due to inadequate absorption but the cause of the latter is not certain. The most likely explanation is the rapid rate of passage of food through the upper part of the small intestine that is known to occur following gastrectomy. As iron is absorbed in the jejunum, the rapid passage reduces the time available for release of iron from food protein and its subsequent absorption. Bleeding from the mucosal remnant of the stomach has also been observed, sometimes at a rate of over 150 ml of blood per month (Holt *et al*. 1970).

The malabsorption syndrome is also frequently associated with iron deficiency and many patients present in this manner. They are diagnosed as simple iron deficiency and are treated with oral iron; it is only when they fail to respond that the underlying disease is discovered.

Clinical presentation

Symptoms
A reduction in the oxygen-carrying capacity of the blood might be expected to cause symptoms referable to the cardiovascular and nervous system, and various text-books have suggested the following: malaise, fatigue, faintness, lack of concentration, dizziness, irritability, headache, palpitations, breathlessness, swelling of ankles and pain in the chest. However, these symptoms can clearly be caused by a great variety of other diseases and are common in neurosis. Berry & Nash (1954) have shown that this type of symptom is common in people without anaemia and conversely many people with anaemia do not have symptoms. Berry & Nash found that the incidence of anaemia in women who stated that they were fit and were not tired or breathless was the same (13·8% anaemic) as the incidence in those who complained that they were not fit and were always tired and breathless (12·9% anaemic). There was evidence, however, that the incidence of symptoms was slightly higher in those few people who had haemoglobin values below 10 g/dl. Thus, these symptoms may be due to anaemia in a small number of people and their elicitation in a clinical history requires that a haemoglobin estimation should be carried out. Many patients with iron-deficiency anaemia are, however, without symptoms.

Dysphagia and iron deficiency
For many years the symptom of post-cricoid dysphagia associated in some cases with a web or stricture, has been linked with a hypochromic anaemia and the presence of the two together has been known as the Paterson–Kelly syndrome. Since the hypochromic anaemia in some of the patients with dysphagia was thought to be due to iron deficiency, it came to be generally held that

the iron deficiency was the cause of the dysphagia. More recent evidence has indicated that this is not so (Jacobs & Kilpatrick 1964). Elwood *et al.* (1964a) studied the incidence of post-cricoid dysphagia in people living in the Rhondda Fach and found dysphagia in 1% of males and 5% of females over the age of 45 years. To their surprise, the incidence of anaemia and of iron-deficiency in those patients with dysphagia was the same as in carefully matched control patients without dysphagia, indicating that iron deficiency is not an aetiological factor. Nevertheless, about half the patients who have a sufficiently severe dysphagia to warrant hospital admission have hypochromic anaemia with low serum iron levels (Jacobs & Kilpatrick 1964). Thus, present evidence suggests that iron deficiency is not an aetiological factor in post-cricoid dysphagia, but that when it is present it is secondary either to the reduction in food intake resulting from the dysphagia, or to the achlorhydria which is frequently found in this condition.

Signs
Beveridge *et al.* (1965) reported the incidence of signs associated with iron deficiency to be: redness of tongue and loss of papillae (39%); abnormal nails (flat or spoon-shaped) (28%); angular stomatitis (14%); splenomegaly (11%). Splenic enlargement is not great and normally only the tip of the spleen is felt.

Haematological changes
If iron loss continues after body stores are depleted, then there is insufficient iron to maintain a normal total red cell mass and the haemoglobin concentration falls. There is a progression of changes in the peripheral blood (see p. 157 for methods of estimation). First, the haemoglobin concentration falls below the normal level for the subject. At the same time, the red cells themselves become microcytic, as shown by a fall in mean cell volume (MCV) and this is accompanied by a similar fall in the amount of haemoglobin in each cell (mean cell haemoglobin, MCH). The concentration of haemoglobin in each cell (MCHC) is thus unchanged initially, and the cells are normochromic. It is only in the later stages that the haemoglobin concentration in the cells is reduced and the cells become hypochromic. This is exemplified by the observations of Beutler (1959) that 19 out of 80 patients with iron deficiency anaemia had an MCHC within the normal range of 30–35 g/dl. It was only when the haemoglobin concentration fell below 7 g/dl in

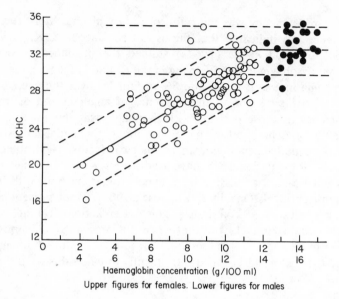

Fig. 1.3. The relationship between MCHC and the haemoglobin concentration in 80 iron deficient (○) and 25 normal subjects (●). Redrawn from Beutler (1959).

women and 9 g/dl in men that the MCHC always fell below the normal range (Fig. 1.3).

On examination of a peripheral blood film, many patients are found to have red cells with a reduced diameter (indicative of microcytosis) and showing variation in size (anisocytosis) and shape (Plate 1b). Accurate assessment of these characteristics by microscopy is, however, subjective. Beutler (1959) showed four blood films made from patients with iron deficiency anaemia to 7 trained haematologists and only obtained complete agreement about the morphological appearances on one of the slides. Nevertheless, microscopic examination of the peripheral blood is very valuable and no haematological diagnosis can be made without it.

Serum iron

Care must be taken in the interpretation of serum-iron concentration in the diagnosis of iron-deficiency anaemia, because there is such a wide fluctuation in the normal values. Average values are 22 µmol/l for males and 20 µmol/l for females, but there is a large

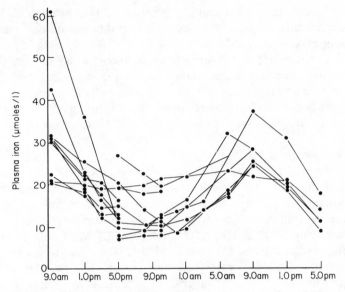

Fig. 1.4. The diurnal variation in the plasma iron concentration of 19 normal individuals. Redrawn from Hamilton *et al.* (1950).

diurnal variation which in males can be as great as between 50 μmol/l in the morning and 10 μmol/l in the evening (Fig. 1.4) (Hamilton *et al.* 1950). Women show a pronounced fall during menstruation and the fall may be as low as 3·5 μmol/l (Zilva & Patston 1966). However, when the haemoglobin concentration falls below 9 g/dl in iron deficiency, the serum-iron concentration is usually consistently below 10 μmol/l (Beutler *et al.* 1958). Conversely a high serum-iron value with a haemoglobin concentration below 9 g/dl probably excludes iron deficiency.

Total iron binding capacity (TIBC) and transferrin saturation
The total amount of iron that can be bound to plasma transferrin usually falls in the range of 50–70 μmol/l plasma. In iron deficiency anaemia the iron-binding capacity is invariably raised when the haemoglobin concentration falls below 9 g/dl and is often raised when the haemoglobin is in the range 9–11 g/dl. Thus, a raised TIBC is a useful diagnostic criterion, although the finding of raised levels in those taking oral contraceptives reduces its value considerably. TIBC is frequently reduced below normal in infec-

tions, neoplasm and rheumatoid arthritis and thus helps to distinguish anaemia in these diseases from that due to iron deficiency (Bainton & Finch 1964).

The percentage of transferrin that is bound with iron (i.e. the ratio of serum iron concentration to total iron-binding capacity expressed as a percentage) is a very useful index for the diagnosis of iron depletion. It has been found that a value of 16% or lower for the transferrin saturation indicates lack of iron stores.

Serum ferritin levels

Ferritin is the major tissue protein for iron storage but is also found in very low concentrations in the serum. Sensitive immunological assays have now been developed for assessing serum ferritin levels and it has been shown that there is a direct relationship between serum ferritin levels and the amount of iron stored in the marrow (Walters *et al*. 1973). Although this test is more complicated to carry out than serum iron and transferrin saturation assays, it is far superior to other tests in differentiating the anaemia resulting from iron deficiency from that due to chronic disease, as short-term physiological variations are much smaller than those seen with plasma iron concentrations. Each 1 μg/l of ferritin in the plasma indicates that there are about 10 mg of stored iron. Thus, a plasma level of 100 μg/l represents a store of 1000 mg of iron. In the absence of iron stores, the plasma ferritin level is less than 12 μg/l.

Even serum ferritin levels may not be a completely reliable guide to iron store levels. Sometimes patients are found with serum ferritin levels above 12 μg/l but who have no stainable iron on bone marrow biopsy. The latter finding may be due to a sampling error, but there are other indications that acute and chronic infections and malignancies may raise serum ferritin levels above that expected from the amount of storage iron.

Free erythrocyte protoporphyrin

Another useful index of iron stores is the presence of the free porphyrin ring in erythrocytes. When iron is not available for inserting into the ring to form haem, the concentration of the iron-free protoporphyrin rises above the upper limit of normal of 70 μg/100 ml of red cell mass. Its usefulness is limited by the fact that it is also raised in the anaemias of chronic diseases in the presence of iron stores.

Measurement of iron absorption

Some patients who are diagnosed as having iron deficiency do not respond to adequate oral iron and it may be necessary to measure the extent of iron absorption, by giving a small standard dose of radioactive ferric chloride (^{59}Fe) to a fasting patient and measuring excretion in the faeces. The amount absorbed is the difference between intake and excretion. Normally the amount absorbed under these conditions is in the range 5–30%. This value is higher than the percentage absorption of iron present in food since, under the radioactive test conditions, the iron is readily available in a soluble form and the patient is fasting, whereas the iron in food is combined to protein and is thus not so readily available.

In iron deficiency, iron absorption is stimulated and the amount absorbed is usually above 50%. Patients who are found to have an iron-deficient anaemia but who have not responded by increasing iron absorption (i.e. iron absorption remains at less than 10% when measured by one of the radioactive techniques), probably have intestinal malabsorption (Badenoch & Callender 1960).

Diagnosis of iron depletion without anaemia

Iron depletion without anaemia can be defined as a state in which there is biochemical evidence of iron lack but haemoglobin concentrations are within the normal limits. The biochemical tests likely to be abnormal are: a decreased serum iron and an increase in total iron binding capacity (i.e. a low transferrin saturation); a

Table 1.1 Changes in measurements of iron status in normal people, patients with iron depletion without anaemia, and in iron deficiency

	Normal	Iron depletion without anaemia	Iron deficiency
Serum iron	10–30 μmol/l	<10	<10
Transferrin iron binding capacity	50–70 μmol/l	>70	>70
Transferrin saturation	>16%	<16%	<16%
Serum ferritin	12–150 μg/l	<12	<12
rbc protoporphyrin	<70 μg/dl	>100	>100
Hb concentration	within normal range	within normal range	below normal range

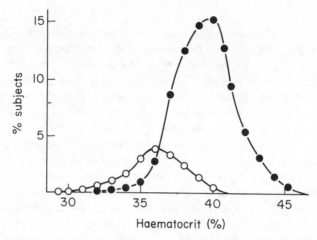

Fig. 1.5. Haemotocrit values obtained from Swedish women before they took 60 mg of iron daily for 3 months: ●——● women who showed no change in haematocrit; ○——○ women whose haematocrit increased in response to the iron therapy. Note that a substantial number of the women whose haematocrit was above the generally accepted lower limit of normal of 35% showed a response to iron therapy. Redrawn from Garby *et al*. (1969).

low plasma ferritin and an increase in red cell protoporphyrin (Table 1.1). As has been emphasized, none of these tests are completely reliable, especially single serum iron measurements, but the probability of detecting iron depletion increases with the number of investigations that yield positive results.

Although the haemoglobin concentration may be within the generally accepted normal range, the value may be below the normal value for that person when iron stores are adequate. To illustrate this, Garby *et al*. (1969) gave iron supplements to a group of apparently normal women and found that a substantial number whose PCV was above the accepted lower limit of 35% showed a rise in haematocrit value (Fig. 1.5).

Treatment of iron-deficiency anaemia

Treatment should start with the oral administration of ferrous sulphate (600 mg $FeSO_4$ containing 120 mg of elemental iron daily, divided into 3-daily doses) as this is the easiest, cheapest and safest method. Stevens (1958) found that the minimal response in iron-deficient patients was a rise in haemoglobin concentration of 2 g/dl in 3 weeks (Fig. 1.6) and most had rates considerably in

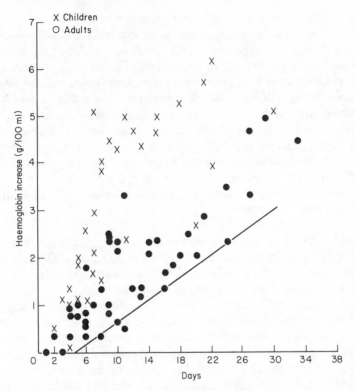

Fig. 1.6. Blood regeneration following intramuscular iron therapy. The minimal response of iron-deficient patients is indicated as a straight line intersecting 2 g/100 ml haemoglobin increase at 21 days. Children responded much faster than adults. Provided the iron is absorbed, oral iron produces as rapid a response as intramuscular iron. Redrawn from Stevens (1958).

excess of this. The haemoglobin concentration of the patient should therefore be measured again 3 weeks later to determine whether there has been an adequate response. If the patient has not responded the following should be considered.

1   That the patient has not taken the tablets. About one-third of antenatal patients in hospital and general practice were found not to be taking the iron tablets which had been prescribed for them (Afifi *et al.* 1966). The authors pointed out that if the incidence held throughout the country, then this would represent a wastage of iron equivalent to 8 small motor cars each year. One of the common reasons for not taking iron tablets is that the patient

claims that they cause gastrointestinal symptoms, such as pain, diarrhoea or constipation. There is undoubtedly a psychological element in these symptoms since Girdwood (1952) found that when ferrous sulphate given as green pills caused symptoms, these disappeared when white pills were substituted. Those patients who cannot tolerate ferrous sulphate, whatever the cause, should be given another iron compound (e.g. ferrous gluconate, etc.).

2 That the patient has the malabsorption syndrome. Patients with this syndrome often present with iron-deficiency anaemia.

3 If the iron deficiency was due to haemorrhage, this may still be operative, e.g. continued bleeding from the gut.

4 That the inital diagnosis was incorrect, or that B_{12} or folate deficiency is also present.

The purpose of treatment with iron is not only to restore the red cell volume to normal but also to replenish iron stores. The former is easy but the latter is difficult. If the patient absorbs only 10% of the 120 mg iron ingested each day as ferrous sulphate, then it will take approximately 3 months to raise iron stores to approximately 1 g. In practice it has been found that the percentage of iron absorbed is often less than this and the patient should therefore be persuaded to continue taking iron for 6 months. The failure rate with oral iron therapy is high. Fry (1961) found that 32% of his patients with iron-deficiency anaemia were still anaemic 5–10 years later. Perhaps these were the one-third of patients who did not take their iron tablets.

Patients with a gastrectomy relapse so frequently after a single course of iron that it has been recommended that they should be given continuous therapy at 200 mg ferrous sulphate a day (Tovey & Clark 1980).

Patients with the malabsorption syndrome and those who cannot tolerate any form of iron orally, should be given iron parenterally. The safest preparations are those which are given intramuscularly. The dose can be calculated approximately from the extent of the anaemia. Thus, a patient with a haemoglobin concentration of 7 g/dl will have a᾽ red cell volume of 100 ml (half the normal value). That is to say, 1000 mg of iron must be given to restore the red-cell volume (1 ml cells contains 1 mg iron), and a further 1000 mg are given to restore iron stores.

The intramuscular preparations, such as iron-dextran, contain iron bound in colloidal form to a carbohydrate compound. The colloidal form does not ionize, so it does not cause toxic symptoms. The colloidal particles reach the circulation and are removed by reticuloendothelial cells. The rate of response in the rise in haemoglobin concentration is not faster with parenteral iron than with oral iron, so that there is no advantage in giving this form of therapy if a quick response is required.

The total amount of iron required for treatment can be given as iron-dextran intravenously, diluted in a large volume of saline and infused over 8–10 hours. Systemic reactions, such as headache, fever, nausea and joint pains are common.

It has been stated (p. 7) that iron stores are usually absent in pregnancy, but there is controversy as to whether all pregnant women should be treated with iron irrespective of their haemoglobin concentration or only when the haemoglobin falls below an arbitrary value (such as 11·0 g/dl, see p. 157). The argument against treating all pregnant women with iron is that when this is done, haematological investigations are often omitted, so that other causes of anaemia (such as folate deficiency) are missed. Moreover, a considerable proportion of patients do not take the prescribed tablets, nor is the obstetrician informed of this. Many are of the opinion that it is safest to estimate the haemoglobin concentration frequently and prescribe iron when required (Verloop 1970).

Anaemias in chronic disorders

The commonest type of anaemia seen in hospital in-patients is that associated with chronic disorders, such as chronic infections, neoplasia, rheumatoid arthritis, renal failure and a large number of rarer disorders. The characteristic findings are as follows:

1 A mild degree of anaemia: commonly the red cells are unchanged in morphology; less commonly, there is some hypochromia present and occasionally both hypochromia and microcytosis.
2 A low serum iron concentration, a low total iron-binding capacity (TIBC) and a reduced transferrin saturation; iron stores are present in the marrow.

The anaemia usually develops within the first 2 months of the disease and then stabilizes at a fairly constant level. The anaemia must be distinguished from iron lack, since it does not respond to iron therapy. The only certain way of making the differential diagnosis is to demonstrate the presence or absence of iron stores in the marrow, but this is not a practical procedure in an anaemia which is so common. The simplest and best of the available tests is a determination of the serum ferritin concentration, which gives a very reliable estimate of the extent of iron stores and will be found to lie within normal limits. Estimation of the total iron-binding capacity can be helpful, since it is often below the normal range in the anaemia of chronic diseases, and frequently above it in iron deficiency. If it is found to be within the normal range, then it does not provide help in the diagnosis. The degree of microcytosis is sometimes useful, since if it is below 70 fl, then iron deficiency is almost certainly present.

The cause of the anaemia is not yet well-defined, but 3 factors have been established.

1 The most important cause is a failure of erythropoietin production, especially in response to a falling haemoglobin concentration.
2 There is a decrease in the life span of the red cells due to extracorpuscular factors.
3 There is a failure to release iron from stores for new red-cell production (Cartwright & Lee 1971).

References

AFIFI A. M. *et al*. (1966) Simple test for ingested iron in hospital and domiciliary practice. *Brit. med. J.*, **1**, 1021.

AISEN P. (1982) Current concepts in iron metabolism. *Clinics in Haematology*, **11**, 241.

BADENOCH J. & CALLENDER, S. T. (1960) Effect of corticosteroids and gluten-free diet on absorption of iron in idiopathic steatorrhoea and coeliac disease. *Lancet*, **i**, 192.

BAINTON D. F. & FINCH C. A. (1984) Diagnosis of iron deficiency. *Am. J. Med.*, **37**, 62.

BENTLEY D. P. & WILLIAMS P. (1974) Serum ferritin concentrations as an index of storage iron in rheumatoid arthritis. *J. clin. Path.*, **27**, 786.

BERRY W. T. C. & NASH F. A. (1954) Symptoms as a guide to anaemia. *Brit. med. J.*, **1**, 918.

BEUTLER E. (1959) Red cell indices in the diagnosis of iron deficiency anaemia. *Ann. Int. Med.*, **50**, 313.

BEUTLER E., ROBSON M. J. & BUTTENWEISER E. (1958) A comparison of plasma iron, iron-binding capacity, sternal marrow iron and other methods in the clinical evaluation of iron stores. *Ann. Int. Med.*, **48**, 60.

BEUTLER E., LARSH S. E. & GURNEY C. W. (1960) Iron therapy in chronically fatigued non-anaemic women: a double-blind study. *Ann. Int. Med.*, **52**, 378.

BEVERIDGE B. R., BANNERMAN R. M., EVANSON J. M. & WITTS L. J. (1965) Hypochromic anaemia. *Quart. J. Med.*, **34**, 145.

BOTHWELL T. H. (1968) The control of iron absorption. *Brit. J. Haemat.*, **14**, 453.

BOTHWELL T. H. & FINCH C. A. (1962) *Iron Metabolism*. Churchill, London.

BRUMFITT W. (1960) Primary iron-deficiency anaemia in young men. *Quart. J. Med.*, **29**, 1.

BURMAN D. (1982) Iron deficiency in infants and childhood. *Clinics in Haematology*, **11**, 339.

CARTWRIGHT G. E. & LEE G. R. (1971) The anaemia of chronic disorders. Annotation *Brit. J. Haemat.*, **21**, 147.

CHANARIN I. & ROTHMAN, DOREEN (1965) Iron deficiency and its relation to folic-acid status in pregnancy: Results of a clinical trial. *Brit. med. J.*, **1**, 480.

COOK J. D. and 13 others (1971) Nutritional deficiency and anaemia in Latin America. *Blood*, **38**, 591.

COOK J. D., FINCH C. A. and SMITH N. J. (1976) Evaluation of the iron status of a population. *Blood*, **48**, 449.

DAVIS L. R., MARTEN R. H. & SARKANY I. (1960) Iron-deficiency anaemia in European and West Indian infants in London. *Brit. med. J.*, **2**, 1426–8.

ELWOOD P. C., JACOBS A., PITMAN R. G. & ENTWHISTLE C. C. (1964a) Epidemiology of the Paterson-Kelly syndrome. *Lancet*, **ii**, 716.

ELWOOD P. C., WITHEY J. L. & KILPATRICK G. S. (1964b) Distribution of haemoglobin level in a group of schoolchildren and its relation to height, weight, and other variables. *Brit. J. Prev. Soc. Med.*, **18**, 125.

FINCH C. A. & LODEN, BETTY (1959) Body iron exchange in man. *J. clin. Invest.* **38**, 392.

FRY J. (1961) Clinical patterns and course of anaemia in general practice. *Brit. med. J.*, **2**, 1732.

GARBY L., IONELL L. & WERNER I. (1969) Iron deficiency in women of fertile age in a Swedish community. *Acta Med. Scand.*, **185**, 113.

GILES C. & BURTON H. (1960) Observation on prevention and diagnosis of anaemia in pregnancy. *Brit. med. J.*, **2**, 636.

GIRDWOOD R. H. (1952) Treatment of anaemia. *Brit. med. J.*, **1**, 599.

GOLDBERG A., LOCHHEAD ANNE C. & DAGG J. H. (1963) Histamine-fast achlorhydria and iron absorption. *Lancet*, **i**, 848.

HALBERG L., HÖOGDAHT A. M., NILSSON L. & RYBO G. (1966) Menstrual blood loss and iron deficiency. *Acta med. Scand.*, **180**, 639–50.

HAMILTON L. D., GUBLER C. J., CARTWRIGHT G. E. & WINTROBE M. M. (1950) Diurnal variation in the plasma iron level of Man. *Proc. Soc. exp. Biol. Med.*, **75**, 65.

HOLT J. M., GEAR M. W. L. & WARNER G. T. (1970) The role of chronic blood loss in the pathogenesis of postgastrectomy iron-deficiency anaemia. *Gut*, **11**, 847.

JACOBS A. & KILPATRICK G. S. (1964) The Paterson–Kelly syndrome. *Brit. med. J.*, **2**, 79.

JACOBS A., KILPATRICK G. S. & WITHEY J. L. (1965) Iron-deficiency anaemia in adults, prevalence and prevention. *Postgrad. med. J.*, **41**, 418.

JACOBS A., WATERS W. E., CAMPBELL H. & BARROW A. (1969) A random sample from Wales. *Brit. J. Haemat.*, **17**, 581.

SCOTT D. E. I PRITCHARD J. A. (1967) Iron deficiency in healthy college women. *J. Am. med. Ass.*, **199**, 897.

STEVENS A. R. (1958) In *Iron in Clinical Medicine* (eds R. O. Wallerstein & S. R. Mettler). University of California Press.

TOVEY F. I. & CLARK C. G. (1980) Anaemia after partial gastrectomy: a neglected curable condition. *Lancet* **i**, 956.

VERLOOP M. C. (1970) Iron depletion without anaemia: a controversial subject. *Blood*, **36**, 657.

VITERI F. E. & TORUN B. (1974) Anaemia and physical work capacity. *Clinics in Haematology*, **3**, 609.

WALTERS G. O., MILLER F. M. & WORWOOD M. (1973) Serum ferritin concentrations and iron stores in normal subjects. *J. clin. Path.*, **26**, 770.

ZILVA J. F. & PATSTON V. J. (1966) Variation in serum-iron in healthy women. *Lancet*, **i**, 459–62.

Objectives in learning: iron deficiency

1   To know the mechanisms concerned in the absorption of iron, its site of storage, method of plasma transportation, and mechanism and extent of loss in men and women.

2   To classify and to know about the causes of iron deficiency at all ages and in both sexes.

3   To know the mode of presentation of iron-deficiency anaemia.

4   To know the changes in red cells indices, in the morphology of the red cells, in the plasma iron levels, and in the marrow histology associated with iron deficiency.

5   To differentiate between the anaemia of chronic infection or neoplasm and that due to iron deficiency.

6   To know the principle of treatment, both by the oral and parenteral routes.

Chapter 2
Megaloblastic, Macrocytic Anaemias

Vitamin B_{12} and folate deficiencies

Deficiencies of both vitamin B_{12} and folate produce identical changes in cell morphology in the bone marrow and in the peripheral blood. It is useful to classify the changes under the heading of megaloblastic and macrocytic anaemia, as the finding of megaloblasts in the bone marrow and of macrocytic cells in the circulation are of prime importance in the diagnosis of these diseases. Folate and B_{12} (Fig. 2.1) are concerned with purine and pyrimidine synthesis and hence with the production of deoxyribosenucleic acid (DNA) and ribosenucleic acid (RNA). Deficiency of either folate or B_{12} leads to abnormalities in the morphology of cell nuclei which are most easily recognized in the red-cell precursors obtained by bone marrow biopsy. The abnormal red-cell precursors, known as megaloblasts, are larger and have a much finer reticular structure of the nucleus than normal red-cell precursors (Plate 3). The increase in size of the megaloblasts persists in the mature red cell, so that the cells found in the peripheral blood are macrocytic.

Macrocytic red cells have in the past been described in certain patients who were suffering from liver disease, hypothyroidism, haemolytic anaemias, Hodgkin's disease, myelosclerosis and tuberculosis. It is now realized that many of these patients probably had either folate or B_{12} deficiency and the finding of macrocytic red cells should always be followed by an assessment of B_{12} and folate stores.

Vitamin B_{12} deficiency

Vitamin B_{12} was among the last of the B vitamins to be isolated; little is as yet known about its biochemical functions. Like the other B vitamins, it acts as a co-enzyme in several enzymatic reactions. It is concerned, together with folic acid, in the transfer of methyl groups in the synthesis of methionine (Fig. 2.2). It has been

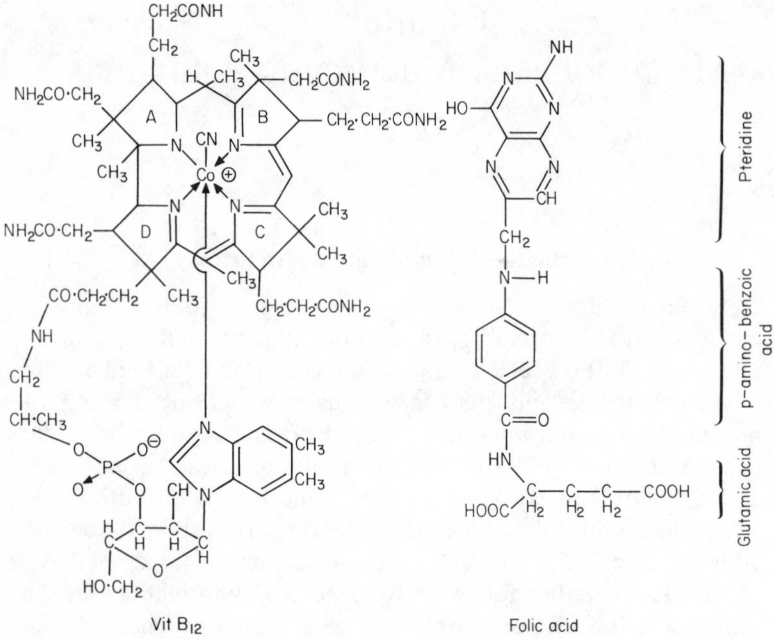

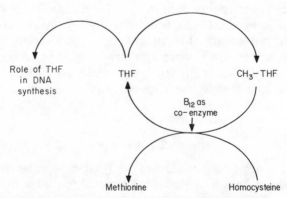

Fig. 2.1. The structure of vitamin B_{12} and folic acid.

Fig. 2.2. The metabolic interrelationship between B_{12} and folic acid and derivatives. Methyl-tetrahydrofolate (CH_3–THF) transfers a methyl group to homocysteine to form methionine. It is this step which requires B_{12} as a coenzyme.

suggested that the reason why deficiency of B_{12} and folate both give a megaloblastic bone marrow is the failure of this metabolic step, in which both are concerned. As can be seen from Fig. 2.2, a lack of either methyl-tetrahydrofolate or B_{12} results in a lack of tetrahydrofolate (THF) and this lack in turn results in a failure of DNA synthesis. The exact role of THF in DNA synthesis has not yet been defined, but it is possible that a deficiency of THF may result in a failure of production of the DNA precursor thymidine triphosphate. Vitamin B_{12} may also play an essential role in the general utilization of amino-acids for protein biosynthesis. Although vitamin B_{12} is required for the proper functioning of every cell, signs and symptoms of deficiency are usually referable to the haematological, gastrointestinal and neurological systems.

B_{12} in the diet. Vitamin B_{12} is produced entirely by bacteria and none is present in plants. Herbivora obtain vitamin B_{12} mainly as the result of synthesis by bacteria in their rumen; other animals and man obtain it by eating animal food. The amount of B_{12} in the diet is usually considerably in excess of the minimum daily requirements for humans.

Mechanism of absorption. Vitamin B_{12} ingested in physiological amounts is not absorbed unless it is first combined with intrinsic factor. The function of this factor is the transport of B_{12} into the epithelial cells of the distal half of the small intestine.

Intrinsic factor is produced in the body of the stomach by the same cells as produce hydrochloric acid, namely, the gastric parietal cells. Chemically, intrinsic factor is a glycoprotein with a molecular weight of about 55,000. The amount of intrinsic factor in the gastric juice can be estimated indirectly by measuring the amount of vitamin B_{12} that it can bind. The amount secreted each day is in the order of 50,000 units. The daily requirement of vitamin B_{12} is about 3–5 μg, and this requires only 3000–5000 units of intrinsic factor for absorption. Thus, the amount of intrinsic factor produced daily is considerably in excess of that required to maintain adequate body stores of vitamin B_{12} (Ardeman & Chanarin 1965).

Storage and rate of loss of vitamin B_{12}. Vitamin B_{12} is mainly stored in the liver and the average healthy adult has a total body content of about 3 mg. Loss of vitamin B_{12} takes place through desqua-

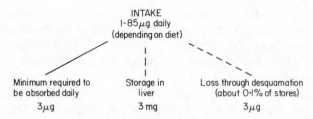

Fig. 2.3. A summary of the absorption, storage and excretion of B_{12}.

mation of epithelium and through excretion in the bile. The rate of loss of vitamin B_{12} is approximately 0·1% of the total body content each day (Fig. 2.3).

Factors causing deficiency

The two commonest causes of B_{12} deficiency are a failure to secrete intrinsic factor and a failure to absorb B_{12} as a result of abnormalities in the ileum. Deficiency resulting from absence of B_{12} in the diet only occurs in strict vegetarians who eat no animal protein at all, although serum B_{12} levels at the lower end of the normal range are commonplace in vegetarians who also eat dairy products.

Failure to secrete intrinsic factor

Intrinsic-factor deficiency is most commonly seen in pernicious anaemia. In England, the prevalence of pernicious anaemia is just over 1 per 1,000 of the population. Approximately 20–30% of all cases have a relative with the disease and this strongly suggests that pernicious anaemia is due to a genetic defect. The nature of the defect is conjectural at the present time. Initially it was suggested that the defect was an inborn susceptibility to the development of gastric atrophy in adult life leading to failure of intrinsic factor secretion, but the recent findings of the presence of serum antibodies against both intrinsic factor and parietal cells has raised the possibility that pernicious anaemia is an autoimmune disease. Antibodies against intrinsic factors are found in about 55% and antibodies against the gastric parietal cell in about 85% of patients with pernicious anaemia. But the fact that they cannot be detected in all cases, combined with the observations that a few patients with thyroid disorders have anti-intrinsic factor antibodies but do not have B_{12} deficiency, suggest that it is not the serum antibodies that are the primary cause of failure of intrinsic factor secretion, although they may play a minor secondary role in decreasing B_{12} uptake. It is possible on the other hand that the gastric atrophy may be the result of cell-mediated immunity (T-cell lymphocyte activity).

Vitamin B_{12} deficiency is also an invariable result of total gastrectomy, provided the patient lives long enough to exhaust his original body stores of B_{12}. Deficiency may also develop after partial gastrectomy but usually not before 5 years have elapsed, and is due to the removal of most of the intrinsic factor-producing area of the stomach and atrophy of the remaining mucosa. The incidence of deficiency after partial gastrectomy is sufficiently high to warrant routine periodic examination of the blood in all patients. Deller & Witts (1962) investigated 285 patients with partial gastrectomy for up to 12 years following the operation and found 54 who were anaemic. In most of the patients the anaemia was due to iron deficiency, but 5% of all the patients examined had evidence of B_{12} deficiency and 2 of the patients had subacute combined degeneration of the cord.

Abnormalities of the small gut
Diversion of B_{12} in the gut can occur due to successful competition by bacteria or by the fish tape-worm, *Diphyllobothrium latum*, which was common in Finland, but is now becoming rare.

Macrocytic anaemia often arises in patients who have anatomical abnormalities of the small gut (blind loops, fistulae, diverticulosis, anastamoses and others) which lead to stasis and bacterial infection. Many strains of bacteria found in these conditions can take up vitamin B_{12}, leaving none for absorption by the host. Folic acid is not affected in this way and in fact folic acid may be produced by the intestinal organisms and thus folic acid stores may be high.

Malabsorption of B_{12} due to disease of the terminal ileum may be seen in coeliac disease and regional ileitis, and is almost invariable in chronic tropical sprue often combined with folic-acid deficiency. There is also reduced absorption after ileal resection.

There is almost always several years delay between the onset of the lesion leading to a failure to absorb B_{12} and the onset of the anaemia resulting from the final disappearance of B_{12} stores. This delay results from two factors. First, intrinsic factor is secreted in considerable excess of the minimum requirement and in pernicious anaemia it takes many years before secretion is reduced to a level when B_{12} absorption becomes inadequate to maintain body stores. Thus, pernicious anaemia almost always develops in the later decades of life. Secondly, since only 0·1% of the body stores of B_{12} are lost each day, it takes several years for the usual body stores of about 3 mg to be reduced to a level (possibly 0·1 mg) which results in megaloblastic anaemia. Following total gastrectomy for instance, it takes about 2–7 years before the B_{12} stores become depleted.

Clinical picture of pernicious anaemia

Pernicious anaemia is not a general term for B_{12} deficiency but refers specifically to adults with severe malabsorption of B_{12} due to a failure to secrete intrinsic factor, secondary to atrophic gastritis. It was first described by Thomas Addison of Guy's Hospital, London, in 1849, and is thus sometimes referred to as Addisonian pernicious anaemia. Diagnosis of pernicious anaemia is only infrequently made on the patient's history and clinical examination alone, the reason being that pernicious anaemia has no specific clinical picture. Pernicious anaemia should not be regarded only as a disease in which there is a deficient production of red cells but rather as a deficiency disease affecting all cells of the body. Signs and symptoms may be mainly referable either to the brain, spinal cord or peripheral nerves, or to the gastrointestinal tract from the tongue down to the colon, or to a failure of bone-marrow activity. The anaemia may also aggravate an underlying cardiac disease.

Davidson (1957) found the four most common presenting symptoms were tiredness and weakness (90% of patients), dyspnoea (70%), paraesthesia (38%) and sore tongue (25%). Although many patients complained of vague intestinal disturbance, diarrhoea only occurred in 9%. Apart from pallor, the most common sign was atrophic glossitis (64%). Commonly, some degree of papillary atrophy of the tongue is seen as an unusual smoothness at the edges, but this sometimes spreads over the entire dorsal surface. It is less common for the tongue to be red, painful and ulcerated. Fever was present in 22% and the spleen was slightly enlarged in only 8% of the cases, and then usually only the tip was felt.

Neurological features appeared in only a small number (7%) of Davidson's patients. The usual syndrome is referred to as subacute combined degeneration of the cord as both the posterior and lateral columns are frequently affected. It is not, however, a satisfactory name, since the onset of the disease is usually insidious and not subacute, lesions of the posterior and lateral columns can occur alone and are not necessarily combined, and the syndrome frequently includes lesions of the peripheral nerves as well as the spinal cord.

Neurologists find it difficult to distinguish with certainty between peripheral neuritis and posterior column involvement, since in both conditions tendon reflexes, vibrational and positional sense may be reduced, and ataxia may be present. However, hyperalgesia of calf muscles favours peripheral neuritis, whereas a disproportionate reduction in positional and vibrational sense up to the pelvis compared to touch and pin-prick favours involvement of the lateral columns. An extensor plantar response indicates pyramidal tract involvement. Individual patients vary as to the extent to which lesions in the posterior columns, lateral columns, or peripheral nerves dominate the neurological syndrome. Central lesions may predominate in the absence of peripheral neuritis and vice versa. Psychiatric symptoms are probably rare, although there is some controversy over this point. Some patients have been rescued from mental institutions and restored to health by B_{12} injections. Neurological involvement may occur without anaemia although the bone marrow usually shows megaloblastic changes.

Davidson concluded that 'there are no pathognomonic symptoms or signs which will establish the diagnosis of pernicious anaemia; that tiredness, breathlessness, paraesthesia and chronic atrophic glossitis are presenting features which occur frequently in other types of anaemia and in particular in cases of iron-deficiency anaemia'.

A study by Hall (1965) also stresses that pernicious anaemia does not have a single typical manner of presentation. The difficulty of making the diagnosis from the initial examination of the patient is shown by his finding that of 40 patients admitted to hospital, in only one was the diagnosis firmly made by the admitting physician.

Seaton & Goldberg (1960) pointed out the similarities between the presenting signs and symptoms seen in pernicious anaemia and those seen in gastric carcinoma. They investigated 50 cases of each disease and found the following clinical features in both pernicious anaemia and gastric carcinoma – lack of energy, pallor, dyspnoea, anorexia, abdominal symptoms and loss of weight. The symptoms referable to the alimentary tract in both groups were epigastric pain or discomfort, heartburn, sour mouthfuls, flatulence, nausea, vomiting and diarrhoea. It was impossible to distinguish between the two diseases on the basis of these clinical features alone. Other features confusing the diagnosis were that some of the patients with pernicious anaemia had occult blood in the faeces and on the other hand one-third of those with carcinoma had histamine-fast achlorhydria; in fact one-fifth of the patients with pernicious anaemia were initially diagnosed as gastric carcinoma.

There is some disagreement about the incidence of weight loss in pernicious anaemia. Seaton & Goldberg (1960) found that a considerable number of patients with pernicious anaemia had a loss of weight of more than 6 kg during the preceding year. This conflicts with the original description of Thomas Addison who emphasized that the patients remained obese. Whatever the true incidence of weight loss, it is clear that the symptom is compatible with pernicious anaemia and does not favour gastric carcinoma. The weight is regained after treatment with B_{12}.

Diagnosis of pernicious anaemia
Witts (1966) has defined pernicious anaemia as a 'megaloblastic anaemia due to defective secretion of intrinsic factor by the stomach which in the adult is always associated with atrophic gastritis or gastric atrophy'. The diagnosis could thus be made by the finding of a macrocytic anaemia together with an assay of intrinsic-factor secretion and a gastric biopsy to demonstrate atrophy. Unfortunately, assay of intrinsic factor and gastric biopsy by suction tube are not routine procedures, and the diagnosis is usually made on other criteria. Intrinsic factor deficiency is more frequently demonstrated by indirect means, i.e. by the demonstration of deficient absorption of radioactive B_{12}. The serum B_{12} level is always low and complete achlorhydria is always present.

Macrocytic anaemia
The average diameter of a red cell is normally within the range 6–8 μm. In a patient with macrocytic anaemia, red cells have an average diameter of about 8–9 μm (Fig. 2.4. and Plate 1). A haematologist viewing many blood smears daily rapidly becomes accustomed to the normal range of red-cell diameters and the eye

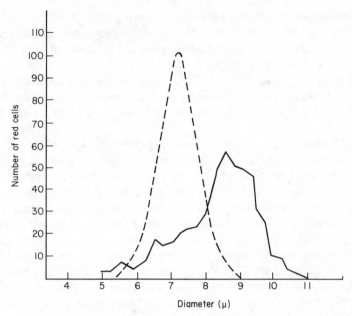

Fig. 2.4. The distribution of the diameter of red cells in microns in a patient with pernicious anaemia (——) compared to the normal distribution (–––).

is quick to appreciate any deviation from the normal. The diagnosis of macrocytosis is thus made in practice on a subjective basis, but it is confirmed by determining the mean corpuscular volume (MCV). This will usually exceed 100 fl.

Examination of a peripheral blood smear also has the advantage that the presence of an excessive number of hypersegmented polymorphs (Plate 4) can be detected. Under normal circumstances, the number of polymorphs with 5 or more lobes does not exceed 3% of the total polymorph population, but in vitamin B_{12} or folic-acid deficiency, an increased percentage of polymorphs with 5 or more lobes is frequently seen and some with 8 or 10 lobes are occasionally present. The presence of hypersegmentation is a useful diagnostic aid although it has recently been realized that hypersegmentation occurs in anaemia due to iron deficiency, and it also occurs in renal failure, even when B_{12} and folate stores are adequate. It is an early sign, although it is usually preceded by marrow changes (Giles 1966).

Megaloblastic changes in the bone marrow
When macrocytic red cells have been found in the peripheral blood, it is usual to proceed with an examination of the bone marrow. The important and characteristic change found in both vitamin B_{12} and folic-acid deficiency is the presence of the megaloblast. The megaloblast is an abnormal red-cell precursor distinguished by its large size and delicate nuclear chromatin, as illustrated in Plate 3.

Another change seen in bone-marrow films which is helpful in making the diagnosis is the presence of giant metamyelocytes, cells which are 2–4 times the normal size and which often have bizarre-shaped nuclei with an abnormal chromatin structure.

Much of the fatty tissue of the marrow is replaced by haemopoietic tissue and microscopically there is considerable hypercellularity. Despite this increased activity, most of the developing red cells do not reach the adult non-nucleated stage but die and are absorbed in the marrow (ineffective erythropoiesis). This failure of maturation is due to a failure of DNA synthesis during division; cells attempt to divide, but do not replicate their DNA content and do not survive.

In severe deficiency of B_{12}, there is also a failure of maturation in the myeloid series of cells and megakaryocytes are also affected, so that there is a deficiency of polymorphs (neutropenia) and thrombocytopenia (Wickramasinghe 1972).

Serum B_{12} concentrations
The diagnosis of B_{12} deficiency can only be made with certainty by the demonstration of the absence of body stores. It has been found that the level of B_{12} in the serum is a reasonably accurate guide to the level of body stores. B_{12} levels can be estimated microbiologically as the organism *Lactobacillus leishmanii* requires B_{12} for growth and reproduction. The organism is incubated in the presence of serum and the extent of growth estimated by the increase in turbidity, which is proportional to the amount of B_{12} present. Extensive investigation has shown that megaloblastic anaemia due to B_{12} deficiency is usually associated with a B_{12} level of below 100 ng/l.

The estimation of serum B_{12} does not, however, give a clear-cut differentiation between abnormal and normal. Low values approaching those seen in B_{12} deficiency are often found in folate deficiency and sometimes in pregnancy and iron deficiency. A few patients with pernicious anaemia substantiated on other grounds have levels which are about 100 ng/l and may be as high as 170 ng/l.

Gastric atrophy and achlorhydria

All cases of pernicious anaemia have a gastric lesion, varying from severe atrophic gastritis to gastric atrophy. As both intrinsic factor and HCl are produced by the same cell, it is perhaps not surprising that achlorhydria is an invariable accompaniment of pernicious anaemia and the diagnosis cannot be made if hydrochloric acid is found to be secreted. The only exceptions to this are cases of congenital intrinsic factor deficiency, when acid secretion is found, but it is possible that the aetiology of the failure of intrinsic factor secretion in the congenital form is different from that of adult pernicious anaemia. Two series of investigations (Callender *et al.* 1960; Wenger *et al.* 1967) have found that the pH of resting juice in pernicious anaemia is usually about 7 and that after maximal stimulation with histamine it does not fall below a pH of 6·0.

Hydrochloric acid is not continuously secreted by the stomach and production must be artificially stimulated before withdrawing gastric juice. Until recently, secretion was stimulated by injecting histamine using the maximal stimulating dose of 0·4 mg/kg; side effects were abolished with antihistamines (the augmented histamine test). Histamine has now been replaced by pentagastrin, the hormone specific for stimulating HCl secretion (Sheaman *et al.* 1967).

Assay of intrinsic factor and vitamin B_{12} absorption

In order to be certain of the diagnosis of pernicious anaemia it is necessary to demonstrate either a marked reduction or the absence of intrinsic factor in gastric juice. A method for assaying intrinsic factor has been described and is being employed to an increasing extent. The method of analysis is the determination of the amount of B_{12} that can be found by constituents of gastric juice. The use of an anti-intrinsic factor antibody can differentiate between the binding of B_{12} by intrinsic factor and the binding by other non-specific binders which do not promote B_{12} absorption (Ardeman & Chanarin 1965).

There is, however, another fundamental test which will demonstrate the failure to absorb B_{12} and will also distinguish between a failure to absorb due to lack of intrinsic factor and those syndromes where the defect lies in the ileum, such as in steatorrhoea. This test is the determination of the extent of absorption of radio-actively labelled B_{12}, as described by Schilling (1953). The test consists of giving 1 μg of $^{57}Co-B_{12}$ by mouth and at the same time 1000 μg of non-radioactive B_{12} is given intramuscularly. This large dose of non-radioactive B_{12} saturates the B_{12}-binding proteins in the plasma and thus causes a substantial proportion of any absorbed $^{57}Co-B_{12}$ to be excreted in the urine. It has been found empirically that B_{12} absorption is impaired when the urinary excre-tion of $^{57}Co-B_{12}$ is less than 10% of that given by mouth, and in pernicious anaemia is almost always below 5%. If the test is abnormal it should be repeated giving both intrinsic factor and $^{57}Co-B_{12}$ by mouth; if the low B_{12} absorption in the patient is the result of intrinsic factor deficiency, then the absorption will be restored to near normal values. This test clearly gives essential information concerning the basic defect and is the most important of all the tests that can be performed.

Treatment of pernicious anaemia

Treatment of patients with pernicious anaemia consists of regular injections of B_{12} for the rest of their lives. A study by Tudhope et al. (1967) has shown that there is a great deal of variation between patients in the length of time that the plasma B_{12} level is main-tained within normal limits following the injection of 500 μg of B_{12}. Thus, 500 μg of cyanocobalamin maintained the plasma level above 100 pg/ml for periods varying between 6 and 54 weeks in the 12 patients examined. In order to take into account those patients whose plasma B_{12} levels fall rapidly, it is necessary to give 250 μg cyanocobalamin every 4 weeks to maintain adequate B_{12} stores. Plasma levels following hydroxycobalamin, however, are maintained for approximately 3 times as long, so that a dose of 1000 μg every 3 months will maintain body stores.

Tudhope et al. (1967) found that 5 of the 12 patients were maintained for at least 1 year after 500 μg of hydroxycobalamin, (Fig. 2.5) and it is thus probably worthwhile finding out which patients can maintain an adequate serum B_{12} concentration after 500–1000 μg every 6–12 months for, although the initial work is increased, a great deal of the patient's and physician's time would be saved subsequently.

It must be emphasized that B_{12} deficiency must never be treated with folic acid alone since, although the anaemia usually responds,

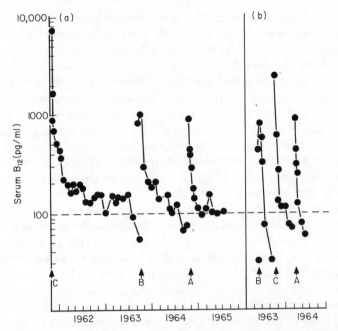

Fig. 2.5. The changes in serum B_{12} concentration after treatment with 500 μg of 3 different forms of vitamin B_{12}: A, cyanocobalamin; B, cyanocobalamin zinc tannate; C, hydroxycobalamin. Note the much lower rate of fall of serum B_{12} in patient (a) compared to (b). From Tudhope *et al.* (1967).

neurological lesions do not and may rapidly progress to an irreversible stage.

Folate deficiency

The commonest cause of megalobalastic anaemia in Britian is pernicious anaemia. Davis & Brown (1953) found that out of 300 consecutive patients with megaloblastic anaemia at Glasgow, 272 had pernicious anaemia. Following the discovery of folic acid in 1941, it was soon realized that many of the remaining patients with megaloblastic changes in fact had folic-acid deficiency.

Folic acid, or pteroylglutamic acid, is composed of three subsidiary molecules, a pteridine nucleus, p-aminobenzoic acid and glutamic acid (Fig. 2.1). Folic acid is required by many plants, bacteria and animals and the success of sulphonamides as a chemotherapeutic agent is dependent on the similarity between the sulphonamide molecule and aminobenzoic acid. Folate-synthesizing bacteria are unable to distinguish between the two molecular forms and sulphonamide blocks folate formation by competitive inhibition.

Folic acid is converted into an active form (tetrahydrofolate) in the body by reduction. The active form acts as a coenzyme in the transfer of single-carbon atom groups (such as formyl, CHO; for-mimino, $CH{=}NH$; and methyl, CH_3) in amino-acid metabolism and in purine and pyrimidine synthesis for the formation of RNA and DNA, and it is probably abnormalities in the latter function which account for the cytological changes in the nucleus characteristic of the megaloblast.

A normal western diet contains about 400 μg of folic acid and the minimum daily requirement is about 100–200 μg in an adult who does not have an increase in metabolic rate or increased turnover of tissue. Absorption is mainly in the duodenum and jejunum and the total body stores are normally about 5–20 mg, greater than the normal body stores of B_{12}. Folic acid is probably degraded enzymatically at the rate of approximately 2% of the total body stores per day, a rate which is 20 times greater than the rate of loss of B_{12}. The rate of degradation is increased when there is increased metabolic activity as in prolonged infection with pyrexia or when there is an increased rate of production of tissue as in haemolytic anaemia and pregnancy. The increased rate of breakdown in these conditions may precipitate folic-acid deficiency.

Clinical presentation

The physiological differences in absorption and metabolism account for the clinical differences in manifestation between folic acid and B_{12} deficiency. B_{12} deficiency mainly results from lack of intrinsic factor or from defects in absorption as in the malabsorption syndrome. As the amount of B_{12} in the diet greatly exceeds the minimal daily requirements, dietary deficiency plays only a minor role in aetiology. On the other hand, as the amount of utilizable folic acid in a normal diet may only be about double the daily requirements, dietary deficiency is one cause of folate deficiency. Malabsorption and an increased rate of turnover are the other two causes.

The more rapid turnover of folic acid compared to B_{12} means that the signs of a folic-acid deficiency appear much sooner than with B_{12} deficiency. Thus, Herbert (1964) found that anaemia developed 5 months after a normal person was put on a folate-deficient diet, whereas it is known that after total gastrectomy, anaemia due to B_{12} deficiency does not develop for 2 years or more.

Megaloblastic anaemia of pregnancy

Megaloblastic anaemia of pregnancy was first described by Channing in 1823 and for a long time was thought to be uncommon, but with the developing interest in folate metabolism it was more diligently sought and found to be relatively common. Megaloblastic anaemia in pregnancy has been well-documented by Giles (1966) who found the incidence to be about 3% of all pregnancies. Out of 1000 patients with haemoglobin concentrations below 10 g/dl, approximately one-third were megaloblastic as judged by bone-marrow biopsy. The more severe the anaemia, the higher the frequency of megaloblastic change so that those patients with haemoglobin levels below 5 g/dl were almost invariably megaloblastic (Fig. 2.6). The highest incidence of megaloblastic change was found within 4 weeks either before or after labour.

The chief cause of folate deficiency in pregnancy is the greatly increased DNA and RNA synthesis associated with the growth of the fetus, placenta and uterus, and the increased red-cell volume of the mother. It has been calculated that folate requirements increase approximately three times during pregnancy (Editorial in *Brit. med.*, 1968). Several subsidiary factors also play a part. Giles found that about one-third of the patients had anorexia and thus presumably a reduced food intake. There also appears to be a reduction in folate absorption during pregnancy, and an increase in folate requirements may result from urinary infection.

Other diseases in which folate deficiency may occur

Folate deficiency and megaloblastic anaemia are found in a variety of diseases where either folate absorption is impaired or where there is increased demand for folate due to increased tissue nucleo-protein metabolism. Concerning malabsorption of folate, deficiency is frequently seen in the malabsorption syndrome where it is also associated with iron deficiency and sometimes with B_{12} deficiency. Failure to absorb folate may also result from inflammation of the gut, as in regional ileitis and from anatomical lesions such as resection of the jejunum, the chief site of absorption.

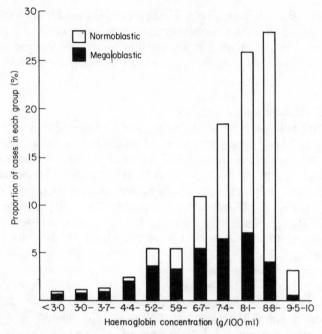

Fig. 2.6. Distribution of haemoglobin levels in 1004 cases of pregnancy anaemia. Note the increasing percentage of megaloblastic anaemia associated with the lower haemoglobin concentrations. From Giles (1966).

Examples of megaloblastic change resulting from increased utilization are infection with sustained pyrexia, and increased red-cell destruction. Thus, the possibility of folate deficiency should always be kept in mind when treating any patient in whom any of these aetiological factors may be occurring.

Diagnosis of folate deficiency
Evidence of folate deficiency can be obtained from the following findings.

1   The presence of anaemia and demonstration of macrocytes in the peripheral blood film.
2   The finding of megaloblasts in the bone marrow.
3   The demonstration of absence of folate stores; unfortunately this assessment cannot be made reliably either from estimates of serum folate or of red-cell folate, although the latter is a more

reliable guide. In practice, therefore, the diagnosis is made on the finding of a macrocytic and megaloblastic anaemia in a patient whose B_{12} stores have been demonstrated to be normal. The diagnosis is then confirmed by showing that the patient responds to a therapeutic trial of folate. Red-cell folate concentrations may be measured and used as confirmatory evidence.

Peripheral blood findings. The most characteristic change found in the peripheral blood is an anaemia with macrocytic cells. However, macrocytic cells are only consistently found when the anaemia is severe. Giles (1966) found that in pregnancy, most patients had normal-sized cells and this was almost always so when the megaloblastic changes in the marrow were minor. Thus, the absence of macrocytes by no means excludes folate deficiency.

Additional evidence of megaloblastic anaemia can be obtained by finding that more than 3% of the polymorphs have 5 or more lobes.

Serum and red-cell folate levels
Lactobacillus casei requires folate compounds for growth, the rate of growth being proportional to the folate content of the media. The concentration of serum folate detected by *L. casei* is not a reliable guide to the state of folate stores, since serum folate levels are sensitive to the dynamic state of folate metabolism; thus, a negative folate balance due to a reduced food intake results in a low-serum folate level within a few days and, according to Chanarin (1969), about one-third of all patients requiring hospital admission in a general hospital have low-serum folate levels. The lower limit of normal for folate varies between laboratories, but most suggest a lower level of 3–4 ng/ml; most patients with megaloblastic changes due to folate deficiency have low-serum folate levels, but exceptions do occur.

Red-cell folate on the other hand is a more reliable guide to folate stores as it is not readily affected by a short period of negative balance of folate. Chanarin (1969) states that patients with normoblastic marrows who have red-cell folate values below normal should be regarded as having folate deficiency. However, in the presence of megaloblastic erythropoiesis red-cell folate is of little use as a diagnostic procedure, since over half the patients with pernicious anaemia have low red-cell folate levels. This probably reflects a true folate defiency, which is secondary to the anorexia so frequently seen in pernicious anaemia, and folate stores return to normal when B_{12} is given. The lower limit of red-cell folate level also varies between laboratories, but a lower limit of 100 ng/ml cells may be taken (Chanarin 1969). Red-cell folate levels are thus a useful guide to the extent of folate stores, but cannot be used alone in the differentiation of B_{12} deficiency from folate deficiency.

Bone-marrow biopsy. Folate deficiency results in an anaemia with megaloblastic changes in the marrow and the diagnosis can only be made confidently by the finding of megaloblasts in the presence of normal B_{12} stores, since identical cytological changes are produced by B_{12} deficiency. It is sometimes possible to avoid doing a bone-marrow biopsy by initially examining a blood film made from the buffy coat, that is from the white-cell layer found on top of the packed red-cell column after centrifuging blood in narrow tubes. Megaloblasts may be found in these films.

Investigation of a patient with suspected folate deficiency
The method of investigation leading to the diagnosis of folate deficiency varies according to the clinical presentation of the patient. In the case of the pregnant woman, the problem is usually the identification of an anaemia which does not respond to oral iron therapy. As iron deficiency is the commonest cause of anaemia in pregnancy, it is reasonable to give oral iron to women with a megaloblastic anaemia the B_{12} status must be fully haemoglobin concentration does not rise and it is established that the patient is taking the iron tablets, then the differential diagnosis usually lies between failure to absorb iron and the presence of folate deficiency. Examination of the peripheral blood and buffy coat for macrocytes, hypersegmentation of polymorphs, and megaloblasts will provide good evidence of folate deficiency, but if a definite diagnosis is required, a sternal marrow biopsy must be carried out. A therapeutic trial with folic acid should then be carried out and if the haemoglobin concentration increases, the reasonable assumption can be made that the patient was deficient in folate.

On the other hand, if a non-pregnant woman or a man presents with a megaloblastic anaemia the B_{12} status must be fully investigated and only if this is found to be normal can folate deficiency be diagnosed. A low red-cell folate level is useful as confirmatory evidence.

Therapeutic trial of B_{12} and folate

The therapeutic trial of either B_{12} or folate is an extremely useful diagnostic tool, if physiological doses of either substance are used. Megaloblastic anaemia due to B_{12} deficiency will respond to 3 μg B_{12} daily by injection but this dose will not affect patients with folate deficiency. Conversely, 200 μg folate daily will cure the megaloblastic anaemia of folate deficiency but will not affect B_{12} deficiency. A haemopoietic response may be followed by observing the reticulocytosis that should reach a peak on the fifth to seventh day (Fig. 2.7). The haemoglobin concentration must be followed until it reaches the normal range, because a few patients, especially those with the malabsorption syndrome, may have a deficiency of both B_{12} and folate, and this can only be definitely revealed by demonstrating that both are required for maintenance of a normal haemoglobin concentration.

If iron deficiency is present at the same time as B_{12} or folate deficiency, the predominant laboratory findings may be either that of iron deficiency or of megaloblastic erythropoiesis and it is only when the predominant feature is corrected by iron, B_{12} or folate that the other deficiency becomes manifest.

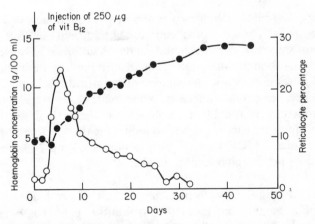

Fig. 2.7. Response of a patient with pernicious anaemia to vitamin B_{12} administration: ●, haemoglobin concentration; ○, reticulocyte percentage.

Treatment

The daily dose of folate depends on the aetiology of the deficiency. The optimal daily dose in pregnancy is still in doubt, but Chanarin *et al.* (1968) have recommended 100 μg starting at the twentieth week and Willoughby & Jewell (1966) give 300 μg during the last trimester (for review, see Editorial in *Brit. med. J.,* 1968). Giles (1966) reduced the incidence of megaloblastic changes to 0·6% by prescribing 5 mg daily. The reason for the failure to eliminate megaloblastic changes with this large dose level is not clear, but could be due to a failure to take the tablets (p. 17). As prescribing folate is not completely effective, haemoglobin estimations must be made throughout pregnancy.

In the malabsorption syndrome, adequate amounts are absorbed if 5 mg are given daily.

Other causes of macrocytosis

With the advent of automatic electronic machines for the estimation of red-cell indices, relatively accurate estimates of MCV have become available on a large number of patients, and it has now become clear that the incidence of macrocytosis not due to B_{12} or folate deficiency is higher than previously thought, one survey finding that 3–4% of patients had large red cells (Davidson & Hamilton 1978). The causes of the macrocytosis are still ill-defined, but there are at least 3 well-documented associations: chronic alcoholism, drugs and hypothyroidism.

Alcohol. Chronic alcoholism is probably the commonest cause of macrocytosis in hospital practice in the U.K. About one-third of a bottle of spirits or its equivalent each day is sufficient to cause the changes. Although folate deficiency, due to inadequate intake, is found in some patients, the majority have neither B_{12} nor folate deficiency, nor are they anaemic. When folate stores are adequate, erythropoiesis is usually normoblastic, not megaloblastic. The macrocytosis appears to be due to a direct toxic affect on red cell erythropoiesis. MCV values return to normal within 2–3 months after stopping the high alcohol intake.

Drugs. Many of the cytotoxic drugs, such as azothioprine and cyclophosphamide, and also anticonvulsants (e.g. the combination of phenobarbitone and phenytoin sodium) affect red cell erythropoiesis and produce megaloblastic changes in the bone marrow and macrocytic red cells. The drugs do not affect B_{12} or folate metabolism.

Hypothyroidism. Macrocytosis has been known to be associated with hypothyroidism for very many years. With the increasing knowledge concerning B_{12} metabolism, it was thought that in almost all cases, the macrocytosis was due to B_{12} deficiency. Indeed, about 10% of all patients with hypothyroidism have pernicious anaemia and both diseases are thought to have similar auto-immune associations. More recent evidence (Horton *et al.* 1976) has shown that the thyroxine deficiency almost always produces a macrocytosis independently of B_{12} and folate deficiency. About one-quarter of all patients with thyroxine deficiency have an MCV above the normal range, and the remainder, although their MCV is within the normal range, all show a fall in MCV of about 10 fl following thyroxine administration.

References

ARDEMAN S. & CHANARIN I. (1965) Assay of gastric intrinsic factor in the diagnosis of Addisonian pernicious anaemia. *Brit. J. Haemat.*, **11**, 305.

CALLENDER S. T., RETIEF F. P. & WITTS L. J. (1960) The augmented histamine test with special reference to achlorhydria. *Gut*, **1**, 326.

CHANARIN I. (1969) *The Megaloblastic Anaemias.* Blackwell Scientific Publications, Oxford.

CHANARIN I., ROTHMAN D., WARD A. & PERRY J. (1968) Folate status and requirment in pregnancy. *Brit. med. J.*, **2**, 390.

DAVIDSON R. J. L. & HAMILTON P. J. (1978) High mean cell volume, its incidence and significance in routine haematology. *J. clin. Path.*, **31**, 395.

DAVIDSON S. (1957) Clinical picture of pernicious anaemia prior to introduction of liver therapy in 1926 and in Edinburgh subsequent to 1944. *Brit. med. J.*, **1**, 241.

DAVIS L. J. & BROWN A. (1953) *The Megaloblastic Anaemias.* Blackwell Scientific Publications, Oxford.

DELLER L. J. & WITTS L. J. (1962) Changes in the blood after partial gastrectomy with special reference to vitamin B_{12}. *Quart. J. Med.*, **31**, 71.

EDITORIAL (1968) Nutritional folate deficiency. *Brit. med. J.*, **2**, 377.

GILES C. (1966) An account of 335 cases of megaloblastic anaemia of pregnancy and puerperium. *J. clin. Path.*, **19**, 1.

HALL C. A. (1965) The nondiagnosis of pernicious anaemia. *Ann. Int. Med.*, **63**, 951.

HERBERT V. (1964) Studies of folate deficiency in man. *Proc. roy. Soc. Med.*, **57**, 377.

HORTON L., COBURN R. J., ENGLAND J. M. & HIMSWORTH R. L. (1976) The haematology of hypothyroidism. *Quart. J. Med.*, **45**, 101.

SCHILLING R. F. (1953) A new test for intrinsic factor activity. *J. lab. clin. Med.*, **42**, 946.

SEATON, D. A. & GOLDBERG A. (1960) Weight-loss in pernicious anaemia. *Lancet*, **i**, 1002.

SHEAMAN D. J. C., FINLAYSON N. D. C., MURRAY-LYON I. M., SAMSON R. R. & GIRDWOOD R. H. (1967) Intrinsic factor secretion in response to pentagastrin. *Lancet*, **ii**, 192.

TUDHOPE G. R., SWAN H. T. & SPRAY G. H. (1967) Patient variation in pernicious anaemia as shown in a clinical trial of cyanocobalamin, hydroxycobalamin and cyanocobalamin–zinc–tannate. *Brit. J. Haemat.*, **13**, 216.

WENGER J., BACKERMAN I., STEINBERG J & GENDEL B. R. (1967) Studies of gastric hydrochloric acid secretion in pernicious anaemia. The value of near maximal stimulation techniques. *Amer. J. Med. Sci.*, **253**, 539.

WICKRAMASINGHE S. N. (1972) Kinetics and morphology of haemopoiesis in pernicious anaemia (Annotation). *Brit. J. Haemat.*, **22**, 111.

WILLOUGHBY M. L. N. & JEWELL F. J. (1966) Investigations of folic acid requirements in pregnancy. *Brit. med. J.*, **2**, 1568.

WITTS L. J. (1966) *The Stomach and Anaemia*. Athlone Press, University of London.

Recommended reading not mentioned in text

CHANARIN I. (1970) Pernicious anaemia and other Vitamin B_{12} deficiency states. *Abst. of World Med.*, **44**, 73.

EDITORIAL (1970) Management of megaloblastic anaemia. *Lancet*, **ii**, 27.

Objectives in learning: the macrocytic anaemias

1 To understand the relationship between the terms macrocytic, megaloblastic, B_{12} deficiency, and folate deficiency.

2 To know the mechanisms of B_{12} and folate absorption, sites of storage and the mechanism and rate of loss of both from the body.

3 To compare and contrast the cause of B_{12} deficiency with folate deficiency.

4 To know the symptoms and signs of pernicious anaemia referable to the gastrointestinal tract, central nervous system, peripheral nerves, cardiovascular and haematological systems.

5 To understand the principles involved in making the diagnosis of pernicious anaemia from an examination of the peripheral blood, bone-marrow biopsy, serum B_{12} levels, extent of absorption of B_{12} and alteration in gastric secretions.

6   To understand the method of differentiation of megaloblastic anaemia due to B_{12} deficiency from that due to folate deficiency.

7   To understand the principle of the therapeutic trial with B_{12} and folate and the principles of treatment with both compounds.

Chapter 3
Haemolytic Anaemias

Under the heading of haemolytic anaemias are grouped a number of diseases which have one abnormality in common, namely, a shortened red-cell life span. Two comments must be made about the term haemolytic anaemia. In the first place, a patient with a diminished red-cell life span is not always anaemic. When there is only a moderate reduction in life span, say 30 days instead of the normal 120 days, a healthy marrow is capable of increasing the rate of red-cell production to maintain the haemoglobin concentration within normal limits. Secondly, the term haemolysis has two meanings in medicine. In the context in which it is used here it means a diminished survival-time of red cells in the circulation. It is also used as a specific term for the process of rupture of the red-cell membrane and release of the cell contents. Intravascular rupture of red cells is rare clinically; in the majority of haemolytic anaemias, the cells of the reticuloendothelial system in either the spleen, liver or bone-marrow remove the red cells from the circulation by phagocytosis.

Haemolytic anaemias are uncommon diseases and in general practice only two or three patients may be seen during a 5-year period (Fry 1961). As haemolytic anaemias are rare, the basic knowledge that is required is concerned with the recognition that a haemolytic process is taking place in a patient. There are a considerable number of diseases which are associated with a haemolytic process and the diagnosis of their precise nature often requires specialized knowledge. The student need only be familiar with those diseases which are most commonly met with. These are: hereditary spherocytosis, the acquired haemolytic anaemias, the commoner haemoglobinopathies (sickle-cell disease and thalassaemia) and glucose-6-phosphate dehydrogenase deficiency (common in certain areas of the world). Those who wish to learn about other haemolytic diseases should consult the monographs of Dacie (1960–67).

Physiology: assessment of rates of red-cell production and destruction

Immature red cells (stem cells, pronormoblasts, basophilic and polychromatic normoblasts, reticulocytes) and adult red cells constitute an organ which is termed the erythron. The primary purpose of the erythron is the exchange of oxygen and carbon dioxide between tissues and environment. This exchange is carried out most efficiently when the ratio of red cells to plasma in the peripheral blood is of the order of 45:55. Lower concentrations of red cells lead to a reduction in oxygen tension in the tissues due to inadequate oxygen-carrying capacity and concentrations higher than this also lead to a reduced oxygen tension due to reduction in the blood flow as a result of increased viscosity.

The maintenance of a constant volume of red cells in the peripheral circulation is the result of a balance between the rates of red-cell production and destruction. The rate of destruction of red cells under normal conditions is fixed by the fact that they are delivered into the circulation with a potential life span of 120 days. Haemorrhage from wounds and from menstrual discharge shorten the life span to a variable extent and the maintenance of a constant and optimum level of red cells is carried out by adjustments in the rate of production through the action of the hormone erythropoietin. Erythropoietin is produced mainly in the kidney, possibly by the juxtaglomerular apparatus, and the amount released is determined by the oxygen tension in that organ. Erythropoietin controls production by increasing the rate of differentiation of the primitive stem cells, by shortening the time of maturation from stem cell to reticulocyte and also by determining the stage at which red cells are released from the marrow; the greater the stimulation by erythropoietin, the earlier the release from the marrow during the reticulocyte stage.

Anaemia is the result of an imbalance between the rates of production and destruction. In most patients, anaemia is due predominantly to a failure of red-cell production, as in iron deficiency, and in only a few patients is excessive red-cell destruction the predominant cause (as in severe haemolytic anaemias).

Red-cell production
In adults, red cells are produced in the marrow at the proximal end of the long bones and in the vertebrae, ribs, sternum, and pelvis. In

the fetus, erythropoietic tissue is found extensively throughout all the bone-marrow and islands of tissue are also found in the liver and spleen. Primary stem cells, which are multipotential, develop into secondary stem cells, which are committed to red-cell production. This secondary stem cell develops into a pronormoblast, a stage which is easily recognized microscopically (Plate 3). After 4 cell divisions, the polychromatic normoblast stage (Plate 3) is reached which is characterized by a small, deeply-staining, amorphous nucleus and abundant cytoplasm. No further division takes place, but haemoglobin is produced within the cell and becomes the predominant component of the cytoplasm, while the nucleus atrophies and the remnants are extruded from the cell. The reticulocyte stage (Plate 3) is characterized by the presence of a cytoplasmic reticulum, demonstrated by staining with supravital dyes before making the blood film. The reticulum is the remains of the ribosenucleic acid (RNA) used in the production of haemoglobin. If the blood film is made first and then stained with the usual haematological stains (such as May–Grünwald–Giemsa), then the RNA does not precipitate as a blue reticulum but remains dispersed, resulting in a red-blue appearance. These cells are termed polychromatic cells and are usually slightly larger than the fully mature adult cell. The final traces of RNA are removed from the red cell during the first 2 days in the circulation. The time of maturation from primitive cell until release as reticulocytes from the marrow is about 5 days, and approximately 20 ml of red cells are produced each day in adults.

When the rate of red-cell destruction is increased, red-cell production in the marrow is stimulated through the erythropoietin mechanism in order to maintain the haemoglobin concentration at the optimal level. In the majority of haemolytic anaemias, the marrow responds to this stimulus and increases the red-cell output. It only fails to do so when there is a lack of iron, B_{12} or folic acid or when the red-cell precursors are damaged or replaced by abnormal tissue, as in leukaemia. If evidence can be obtained of an increased rate of red-cell production above the normal this is good evidence that a haemolytic process is taking place, providing that there has been no loss of red cells through haemorrhage.

Two simple methods are available for assessing whether there is any increase in the rate of formation of red cells, namely, the reticulocyte concentration in the peripheral blood and the erythroid/myeloid ratio in the marrow.

Reticulocyte concentration

After release from the marrow, reticulocytes take 1–2 days to mature into adult red cells. The number of reticulocytes in the peripheral blood is expressed as a percentage of the total number of cells; the normal percentage is usually in the range 0·2–2·0%. Other things being equal, the number of reticulocytes in the circulation should be proportional to the rate of production of red cells, but in practice there is a variation in the length of time that reticulocytes take to mature. For example, the early release of reticulocytes from the marrow following erythropoietin stimulation means that they will spend longer in the circulation before they mature into adult cells. Nevertheless, an increase in the number of reticulocytes is an indication of increased marrow activity and in general, the higher the count, the greater the rate of production of viable red cells delivered to the circulation. Values up to 50% or more of reticulocytes may be obtained when marrow activity is intense.

The erythroid/myeloid ratio

The cells of the erythroid series are normally in a minority in the bone-marrow and the ratio between the erythroid and myeloid series usually varies between 1:3 and 1:15. An increase in the rate of production of red cells is brought about by an increase in the number of red-cell precursors and hence this ratio will increase. When erythroid hyperplasia is marked, this is obvious on visual inspection of a stained bone-marrow biopsy smear when compared to the normal, but where there is doubt an estimate of the erythroid/myeloid ratio can be made. This ratio is, however, of no value if there is concomittant white-cell hyperplasia. A normal peripheral white-cell count and morphology is taken to be evidence that the myeloid series is normal in numbers.

As a result of the simultaneous study of red-cell production and destruction by several different methods (reticulocyte count, erythroid/myeloid ratio, iron turnover, urobilinogen output, red-cell life span), it has become evident that in certain diseases not all developing red cells are finally released into the circulation: instead they are destroyed in the marrow, presumably as a result of malformation. This failure to develop fully is known as ineffective erythropoiesis and is seen particularly in vitamin B_{12} deficiency and thalassaemia. Thus, the finding of hyperplasia of the red-cell precursors in the bone-marrow does not necessarily indicate an increased output of viable cells into the circulation.

Radioactive iron turnover

There is a third method of measuring the activity of the red-cell marrow, which gives a quantitative estimate of total marrow activity, that is, both effective and ineffective erythropoieses. This is the estimation of the total iron turnover in the plasma. The method gives very useful information but requires the use of radioactive iron (^{59}Fe). Under normal conditions, about 30–35 mg of iron pass through the plasma each day. Since 20 ml of red cells are produced each day and as 1 ml of red cells contains approximately 1 mg of iron, 20 mg of the iron passing through the plasma represents that used in production of red cells. The other 10–15 mg of Fe turned over each day represents exchange between stores and tissues other than red-cell precursors. Thus, other things being equal, an increase in iron turnover gives a semi-quantitative index of red-cell precursor activity. An iron turnover of 70 mg/day indicates approximately a two- to three-fold increase in marrow activity.

In certain diseases, the rate of production of red cells can rise to a maximum value of about 6–8 times the normal, that is, to 120–160 ml red cells per day. This is usually seen only in certain haemolytic anaemias, such as hereditary spherocytosis, when the supply of iron from phagocytosed red cells is readily available for new red-cell production. Following haemorrhage, the rate of red-cell production increases to only 2–3 times the normal rate. The upper limit of the rate of production is set by the supply of iron, which is limited by the total plasma flow through the marrow.

Life span and red-cell destruction

The normal red-cell life span is approximately 120 days from the time they enter the peripheral circulation. The cause of their destruction at the end of their life-span is not known. The current hypothesis is that the red cell is delivered to the circulation with a fixed quantity of enzymes associated with energy production from glucose, and that these enzymes are slowly degraded until a level is reached when energy production becomes inadequate to maintain red-cell viability. Approximately 20 ml or 0·85% of the total red-cell mass is destroyed each day. The cells are destroyed by phagocytosis, probably in the spleen, although there is no convincing evidence that this is the site and it is possible that the bone marrow phagocytes may play a significant or even a dominant role.

The extent of the shortening of the red-cell life span in disease varies between individuals and according to the type of disease. In patients with hereditary spherocytosis who have a mild degree of anaemia (e.g. haemoglobin concentration 12–13 g/dl), red-cell survival may only be shortened to 30 days, a value well within the ability of the marrow to compensate (Fig. 3.1). On the other hand, a life span as short as 5 days is sometimes seen in acquired haemolytic anaemia and is always associated with severe anaemia.

Bilirubin metabolism

The simplest method of obtaining evidence for increased red-cell destruction is by estimations of the amount of bilirubin and its derivatives in plasma, faeces and urine. When the red cell is destroyed in the reticuloendothelial cell, the haem is converted into

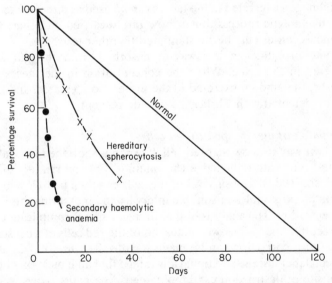

Fig. 3.1. The survival of ^{51}Cr-labelled red cells (corrected for ^{51}Cr elution) in the circulation of: a patient with hereditary spherocytosis (×) whose haemoglobin concentration was 15.5 g/dl, the mean red-cell life span 30 days; and a patient with leukaemia (●), whose haemoglobin concentration was 5 g/dl; the mean red-cell life span 5 days.

bilirubin with the release of carbon monoxide. Free bilirubin is insoluble in water and hence is transported to the liver attached to albumin. In the liver it is converted into the soluble glucuronic acid–bilirubin complex and excreted. There is an upper limit for the rate of complex formation by the liver and, hence, if the supply of bilirubin exceeds this rate, the bilirubin concentration in the plasma rises. Bilirubin concentration therefore does not increase above the normal range if the increased rate of destruction of red cells is only moderate and only begins to rise when the life span is shortened to about 50 days or less. A rise in plasma bilirubin concentration is only significant in the diagnosis of a haemolytic process if liver function is entirely normal.

As far as is known, bilirubin is not catabolized in the body, but excreted in the faeces where it is converted by bacteria into urobilinogen. As an average-sized adult destroys about 20 ml of red cells each day, this should result in the excretion of 200 mg of urobilinogen. When there is an excessive rate of destruction of red cells, the amount of urobilinogen in the faeces rises and causes the faeces to be darker than normal. Estimation of the amount of urobilinogen execreted in the faeces can be used as direct evidence of a haemolytic process, but is now rarely carried out, since the diagnosis can usually be substantiated by other tests.

Some urobilinogen is always reabsorbed from the gut and excreted in the urine. When the concentration in the faeces increases, the amount excreted in the urine also increases, and this can be detected with Ehrlich's aldehyde reagent.

Estimation of the life span of red cells

The best way to show that red-cell life span is shortened is to label the red cells with radioactive chromium (^{51}Cr) and reinject them (Mollison 1983). The survival of the cells can then be followed by taking blood samples at suitable intervals and measuring the ^{51}Cr concentration. The analysis of the survival curve is complicated by the fact that the ^{51}Cr slowly elutes out of the red cells at a constant rate, but a correction can be made for this. The use of ^{51}Cr as a red-cell label has the additional advantage that an indication of the main site of destruction can be obtained. ^{51}Cr emits γ-rays which will penetrate the body tissue and thus ^{51}Cr deposited in the spleen or liver can be detected by placing a γ-ray detector on the surface of the body over these organs. Experience has shown that when the ^{51}Cr accumulates predominantly in the spleen in haemolytic

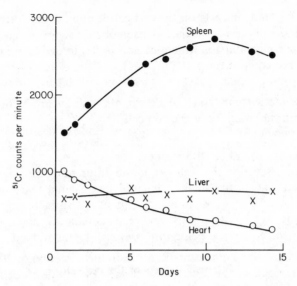

Fig. 3.2. The excessive accumulation of ^{51}Cr in the spleen (●) compared to the counting rate over the liver (×) and heart (○) in a patient with idiopathic autoimmune haemolytic anaemia. Splenectomy in this patient was followed by a complete remission. ^{51}Cr counts obtained from over the spleen in normal people are similar to the counts obtained over the liver.

anaemias, splenectomy is usually followed by a partial or complete cure of the haemolytic process (Fig. 3.2).

Diagnosis of a haemolytic process
The diagnosis of a haemolytic process can be made with reasonable confidence by the finding of an increase in both the reticulocyte count and the plasma bilirubin concentration, provided that other causes for the latter two abnormalities are excluded, e.g. haemorrhage and liver disease. Anaemia may or may not be present. If there is doubt, then estimation of faecal and urinary urobilinogen give very useful confirmatory evidence. The use of ^{51}Cr-labelled red cells requires radioactive counting equipment, but this is now generally available.

The next stage in diagnosis is to determine the nature of the disease which is causing the haemolytic process. In approaching the diagnosis, it is useful to make a distinction between congenital or intrinsic abnormalities of the red cell on the one hand, and acquired or extrinsic abnormalities on the other hand; in the latter category, an agent acts on the red cell leading to its destruction, e.g. autoantibodies in acquired haemolytic anaemia. When considering congenital abnormalities, it is useful to divide the red cell into three component parts:

1 red-cell membrane;
2 enzyme systems concerned with the energy production that maintain the integrity of the red cell;
3 haemoglobin.

Defects are found in all 3 systems.

In the discussion that follows on the different diseases it will be assumed that all the signs of haemolytic anaemia that have just been discussed are present in each patient to a variable degree and only the signs, symptoms and haematological abnormalities specific to the disease being discussed will be mentioned.

Intrinsic defects of the red cell

Red-cell membrane defects

Hereditary spherocytosis
The commonest example of a membrane defect is hereditary spherocytosis, although it may be premature to classify it in this way, since extensive research has so far failed to reveal the precise nature of the abnormality. Recent evidence has suggested that there may be a defect associated with the structural protein, spectrin, which is closely associated with the cytoplasmic surface of the red-cell membrane. This protein may be concerned with the maintenance of the biconcave shape of the red cell and the abnormality may allow the cells to become spherocytes and, in some unknown way, this leads to a reduction in red-cell survival.

The incidence of the disease has been estimated to be 1 per 10,000 of the population in London, so that a large general practice may contain one family with the disease (Mackinney 1965). The disease is transmitted as a dominant genetic defect from either parent. The spontaneous mutation rate is low, so it is usual for patients to be able to give a family history of the condition, such as a parent or sibling who is known to have had the disease or who has had recurrent anaemia, gall stones or a splenectomy.

The disease may present at any time from birth to old age, although it is usually the milder cases who reach adulthood without detection. There is a great difference in the severity of the disease, varying from patients who have a haemoglobin concentration of 4–5 g/dl to patients who are not anaemic at all and who may present only because they have a family history of the disease and desire investigation.

Mackinney (1965) investigated 26 families and found that half the patients had no symptoms but had abnormal findings in the peripheral blood. He also found that half the patients with intact spleens had haemoglobin concentrations of over 12 g/dl.

The rate of destruction of red cells in a particular patient remains fairly constant but the disease is characterized by short periods of exacerbations when the patient becomes more anaemic and frequently develops abdominal pain; in some, jaundice may appear or increase in intensity. This type of crisis which varies in severity from mild to severe, is due to a temporary failure of red-cell production by the bone-marrow. The main evidence for this is a marked fall in the reticulocyte count. A substantial number of these hypoplastic or aplastic crises are associated with a trivial disease such as an upper respiratory tract infection, but it is not known why there is hypoplasia of the erythropoietic tissue. Apart from the failure of red cell production, there may also be an increase in the rate of haemolysis during these crises, thus increasing the degree of anaemia and accounting for the fact that the plasma bilirubin concentration rises. It is common for patients to present for the first time during one of these episodes.

Megaloblastic anaemia due to folate deficiency may also be found, as in other chronic haemolytic disorders. This results from an increased rate of turnover of folate by the hyperactive bone marrow, and is especially found when the diet is inadequate.

Another complication from which these patients suffer, and which is sometimes a presenting symptom, is the development of pigment gall stones. Most patients develop pigment stones, but probably only 10–20% of those with intact spleens develop symptoms sufficiently severe to require cholecystectomy (Mackinney 1965).

Apart from anaemia and jaundice, the main clinical finding in most patients is an enlarged spleen, although this may not be felt in a mild case.

Laboratory investigation. Mackinney (1965) found that there were 4 signs which gave the greatest help in diagnosis: the presence of spherocytes in the stained blood film, an increased reticulocyte count, raised plasma bilirubin, and anaemia. Only a small percentage of the red cells are spherocytes and they appear as small densely staining cells (Plate 2). A further important test which must always be carried out is the demonstration of increased osmotic fragility. Normal red cells do not start to lyse until the saline concentration of the suspending medium is reduced to 0·55 g/dl. In hereditary spherocytosis, the red cells are thicker than normal and some are already spherocytic, so that a fluid uptake smaller than normal is sufficient to burst the cells. Thus, these abnormal cells start to lyse when the saline concentration is reduced to values of only 0·6–0·8 g/dl.

The diagnosis of hereditary spherocytosis is thus made on the basis of a family history, anaemia, raised reticulocyte count and plasma bilirubin concentration, spherocytosis, an increased osmotic fragility and a negative antiglobulin test.

Treatment. The membrane abnormality in hereditary spherocytosis results in increased rigidity of the cells, which do not pass easily through the splenic cords in the red pulp. This leads to stagnation of the circulation and adverse changes in the local environment which, together with the abnormality of the red-cell membrane, results in destruction of the red cells. Splenectomy results in the life span of the cells returning almost to normal.

Enzyme deficiencies causing haemolytic anaemias

The second red-cell compartment in which congenital abnormalities occur is the enzyme system concerned with energy transfer in glucose metabolism. The red cell requires a continuous supply of energy for the maintenance of surface structure, the sodium and potassium pumps and the maintenance of haemoglobin in the reduced ferrous form. The energy is obtained from glucose which is transformed to lactic acid mainly through the anaerobic Embden–Mayerhof pathway. There is an alternative aerobic pathway, the pentose–phosphate shunt, starting with glucose-6-phosphate and requiring glucose-6-phosphate dehydrogenase (G6PD) as the initial enzyme (Fig. 3.3). Energy is transferred through the energy-rich compounds adenosine triphosphate (ATP), nicotinamide-adenine dinucleotide (NADH), the related phosphorylated compound, NADPH, and reduced glutathione (GSH).

The discovery that congenital deficiencies of some of the enzymes concerned with glucose metabolism can occur and give

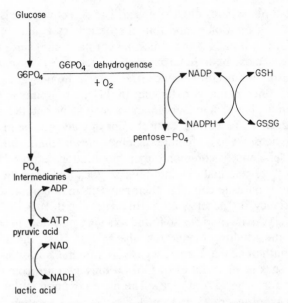

Fig. 3.3. A schematic diagram of the pathway of glucose metabolism in the red cell, to show the important role of glucose-6-PO₄ dehydrogenase. Absence of the enzyme leads to the deficiency of the reducing compounds, NADPH and GSH.

rise to haemolytic anaemia is of fairly recent origin. It was noticed in the decade 1920–30 that the antimalarial drugs, aminoquinolines, produced a haemolytic anaemia in certain individuals, but it was not until the work of Beutler and others (Beutler 1959) that this was found to be a haemolytic anaemia due to a congenital deficiency of glucose-6-phosphate dehydrogenase. At the same time as these investigations were being carried out it was also noticed that there was a type of haemolytic anaemia which could be distinguished from hereditary spherocytosis by the absence of spherocytes and the failure to respond to splenectomy (Haden 1947); it is termed non-spherocytic haemolytic anaemia. It is now known that many of these latter patients have enzyme deficiencies associated with the glycolytic cycle, and the commonest of these deficiencies is absence of G6PD.

Glucose-6-phosphate dehydrogenase deficiency
It has been estimated that there may be as many as a hundred million people in the world who have diminished red-cell concentrations of

glucose-6-phosphate dehydrogenase. The defective gene is present on the X chromosome, and thus the deficiency is mainly seen in males ($\bar{X}Y$, where $\bar{X}$ is the abnormal chromosome) since the normal X chromosome in heterozygous women ($\bar{X}X$) is usually sufficient to maintain G6PD concentration and homozygous women ($\bar{X}\bar{X}$) are uncommon. A deficiency of this nature found in so many people must have some Darwinian survival value and the evidence now indicates that deficiency of the enzyme gives some protection to the heterozygous female against *Plasmodium falciparum*; G6PD deficiency is common only in populations exposed for long periods to tertian malaria and heterozygous females with malaria have lower parasite counts in their red cells than normal women.

Deficiency of the enzyme is found in about 10% of Negroes from West Africa, and is also found to a varying extent in countries around the Mediterranean area, the Middle East, India and the states south of China. Deficiency is very rare in Caucasians. Of the 180 or so known varieties of G6PD, only two are common and account for over 95% of cases. The most common is the African (or A-) type, where G6PD levels are reduced to about 10% of normal; in the less common Mediterranean type, the level is reduced to 1–3% and the resultant anaemia is more severe.

Low concentrations of G6PD results in a low concentration of the reducing compounds NADPH and GSH (Fig. 3.3). The purpose of these compounds is to maintain haemoglobin and other proteins in the reduced and active form. People with low levels of the enzymes are thus poorly protected against drugs which are oxidants. When oxidants enter the red cell they first convert haemoglobin to methaemoglobin and finally denature it so that it precipitates in the red-cell and can be demonstrated as Heinz bodies (p. 164). Other proteins in the red cell are affected in the same way and this results in loss of viability and destruction of the red cells. The formation of Heinz bodies *in vitro* can be used as a screening test for the presence of low concentrations of the enzyme in the red cells. If the drug acetylphenylhydrazine is added to red cells *in vitro* it will cause the formation of a few Heinz bodies in normal people but in those with low concentrations of G6PD many Heinz bodies are formed. The drugs which bring about this type of haemolytic anaemia are the anti-malarial drugs (primaquine and quinine), sulphonamides, analgesics such as aspirin and phenacetin, and other drugs such as vitamin K and quinidine.

Almost all those with low concentrations of G6PD are symptomless under normal conditions and have normal haemoglobin concentrations. There is usually sufficient G6PD to maintain the integrity of the cell, but careful measurement frequently reveals a small degree of shortening of the red-cell life span. Haemolytic anaemia is maximal in these patients about 7–10 days after taking the drug. The extent of the fall in haemoglobin concentration is partly dependent on the amount and nature of the drug being given, but after about 10 days and despite the continuation of the drug the haemoglobin concentration rises again and may reach normal levels. This phenomenon is due to the fact that it is only the older cells in which the G6PD has fallen with age that are affected and destroyed by the drug. Thus, the red-cell life span may be reduced from 120 to 60 days, and this degree of shortening can easily be compensated for by the marrow. Heinz bodies can frequently be demonstrated in the red cells in the circulation during the early stages after administration of the drug.

Very rarely patients may be encountered whose G6PD is so low that it is not possible to maintain the viability of the red cell under normal conditions and a continuous haemolytic process is then present. These patients come into the category of congenital non-spherocytic haemolytic anaemia. This category includes a heterogeneous group of patients, many of whom have G6PD deficiency or a deficiency of other enzymes in the glucose catabolic cycle.

Favism. Favism has been known for 2000 years or more and is now recognized as an acute haemolytic anaemia occurring in those who have both a deficiency of G6PD (only of the Mediterranean type) and also a sensitivity to fava beans. It usually follows ingestion of the beans (*Vicia faba*) but may follow inhalation of the pollen. It usually affects children. The anaemia is rapid and severe and is often accompanied by haemoglobinuria. The factor responsible for the reaction has not been identified.

Haemoglobinopathies

The haemoglobin A molecule (which is the predominant type of molecule in human red cells) is composed of four polypeptide chains, two α and two β chains. These combine together to form a three-dimensional structure, the exact shape of which is critical in maintaining the reversible combination between oxygen and the haem portion of haemoglobin, and also in maintaining the solubility of the haemoglobin molecule within the red cell. An alteration of one of the bases in the genetic DNA responsible for the amino-acid sequence in the polypeptide chains leads to replacement of one amino-acid by another. In many instances this does not alter the function of haemoglobin, but in some instances it does bring about profound changes which result in a shortening of the life span of the red cells.

The commonest example of an abnormal haemoglobin is haemoglobin S, where an uncharged valine molecule is substituted for a charged glutamic acid. This results in an alteration in tertiary structure so that at low-oxygen concentrations, the haemoglobin molecules become more closely and firmly associated together, resulting in the rigid sickle-shaped red cell. If the sickle-shape is maintained for more than a few minutes, the cells remain irreversibly sickled and these cells are rapidly destroyed.

Almost 200 abnormal haemoglobins have been described, but most are extremely rare (Lehmann & Huntsmann 1974). After haemoglobin S, haemoglobin E (occurring in people of south-east Asian extraction) is the next commonest. Haemoglobin C is relatively common in people of West African extraction. Both of these abnormalities are usually seen in the heterozygous state and cause no anaemia, although, target cells (p. 161) are frequently seen. The presence of target cells may be the presenting sign, indicating that the patient has an abnormal haemoglobin. Occasionally the homozygous state is present, when there is usually a mild degree of anaemia secondary to a shortened red-cell survival time. Some abnormalities of the globin molecule affect the oxygen-binding capacity, resulting in a failure to release oxygen, or a failure to bind sufficient oxygen (Hb M) causing cyanosis. Other abnormal haemoglobins (e.g. Hb Köln) are chemically unstable and denature within the red cell, leading to a shortening of red-cell life span.

When the amino-acid substitution results in an overall change in the charge of the molecule, its migration in a voltage gradient is altered and this can be demonstrated by standard electorphoretic techniques. The speed of migration is characteristic for each abnormal haemoglobin (Plate 2).

Haemoglobin S

The gene responsible for Hb S is found to occur in a wide area across tropical Africa, in the Mediterranean, and parts of the Middle

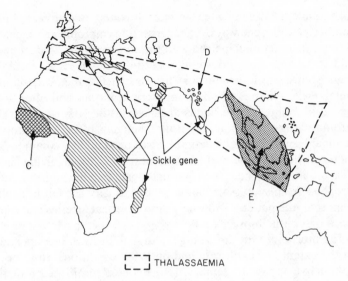

C   D   E   Sickle gene

⌐ ⌐ THALASSAEMIA

Fig. 3.4. Distribution of the major haemoglobin abnormalities (redrawn from Lehmann H. & Ager J. A. M. In Stanbury *et al.* (eds) *The Metabolic Basis of Inherited Disease*. McGraw-Hill, New York, 1960).

East and India (Fig. 3.4). The incidence of the gene varies from very low values up to 40% of the population. In the American negro, the incidence is 10%. The persistence of this potentially lethal gene is due at least in part to the fact that heterozygotes are partially protected during childhood from falciparum malaria. The disease runs a much milder course in the presence of Hb S.

Heterozygotes (one gene for Hb A and one for Hb S) are defined clinically as having sickle-cell trait. Their red cells contain between 20 and 45% Hb S, the rest being mainly Hb A. They are normal haematologically and clinically, although haematuria and splenic infarction can occur under anoxic conditions. The red cells do not sickle in the trait until the oxygen saturation falls below 40%, a level which is rarely reached in venous blood.

Homozygotes for Hb S have sickle-cell anaemia. Their red cells contain 80% or more of Hb S, the remainder being mainly fetal haemoglobin. The cells sickle at the oxygen tension normally found in venous blood (Plate 2). The increased rigidity of the cells causes them to move slowly or even to become jammed in capillaries, with resultant damming-up of blood which eventually leads to infarction.

In infancy and early life, the clinical course is manifested in a number of different ways. The signs and symptoms are those of chronic anaemia interspersed with thrombotic crises. A characteristic feature is dactylitis, or the hand–foot syndrome, resulting from occlusion of the nutrient arteries to the metacarpals and metatarsals. There is a painful, non-erythematous and often symmetrical swelling of the hands and feet, lasting 10–14 days. The thrombotic crises may mimic acute rheumatism or an acute abdominal lesion. In adults, painful crises become less common but leg ulcers become one of the commonest features, involving about 75% of patients. The spleen is usually palpable in children, but it atrophies from successive infarcts and is usually not felt in adults. Almost all the patients show occlusion of retinal arteries and capillaries on ophthalmoscopy.

The mortality rate can be high, although this will be dependent on the extent of health care and on living conditions. In a recent prospective survey in Jamaica (Rogers *et al*. 1978) 13% of the children died in the first 2 years of life. The principle causes of death were acute splenic sequestration of blood and pneumococcal infection, both of extremely rapid onset, but both amenable to treatment. In acute splenic sequestration, there is rapid enlargement of the spleen due to trapped red blood cells and anaemia becomes profound. The reduced blood volume results in hypotension and a state of shock. The condition responds rapidly to transfusion. Bone marrow failure may occur which presents as an aplastic crisis. The cause of the aplasia may be due to folate deficiency and the conversion to megaloblastic erythropoiesis, but is frequently of unknown aetiology.

The diagnosis is made by finding the characteristic sickle cells in the peripheral blood. Under normal conditions, sickle cells are seen in the stained blood-film used for routine microscopy only in those with sickle-cell anaemia. Heterozygotes do not show sickling on the film, unless reducing agents have been added to the blood beforehand. Hb S can also be demonstrated by electrophoresis. Homozygotes have a single main band of haemoglobin S, heterozygotes show a mixture of Hb A and S (Plate 2).

Thalassaemia

Wetherall & Clegg (1981) have defined the thalassaemias as 'a heterogeneous group of genetic disorders of haemoglobin synthesis characterized by imbalanced globin chain production which leads to anaemia, ineffective erythropoiesis and red cell destruction both within the bone marrow and in the peripheral circulation'. The essential difference between the haemoglobinopathies and the thalassaemias is that in the former there are structural changes in the haemoglobin molecule, whereas in the thalassaemias there is a complete or partial failure of synthesis, due either to a failure in mRNA production (β thalassaemias) or to gene deletion (α thalassaemias). The predominant haemoglobin of the adult red cell, Hb A (98% of the total haemoglobin), is composed of 2 α and 2 β chains. Hb A_2 (about 2% of the total adult haemoglobin) has 2 α and 2 δ chains. Fetal haemoglobin (Hb F) has 2 α and 2 γ chains. The thalassaemias are broadly divided into 2 groups, the α thalassaemias and the β thalassaemias, depending on whether the defect lies in the synthesis of α or β chain respectively.

The α-thalassaemias
Under this heading come a heterogenous collection of molecular defects of the α-globin genes which nevertheless result in the expression of similar phenotypes. There are 2 closely-linked α-globin genes on chromosome 16 and thus 4 genes altogether. The severity and manifestations of the disease depend on the number of genes deleted in a particular individual. There are two main varieties of defect. First, one of the two genes on a single chromosome may be deleted (α^+-thalassaemia determinant) or secondly, both genes may be deleted (α^0-thalassaemia determinant). These 2 variants together with the normal genes lead to 5 different combinations (Fig. 3.5).

Deletion of 1 gene. This is seen as a heterozygous state in which the α^+-thalassaemia determinant is present together with a normal chromosome. Patients are either normal or are only slightly anaemic.

Deletion of 2 genes. This arises in 2 ways, either as a homozygous α^+-thalassaemia or as a heterozygous α^0-thalassaemia. Both these combinations give rise to similar mild clinical changes, with a small reduction in haemoglobin concentration.

Deletion of 3 genes. This results from a combination of both the α^+- and α^0-thalassaemia determinants. Only a few α-chains are produced and there is considerable excess of β-chains which combine

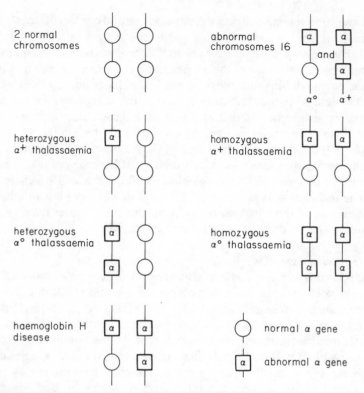

Fig. 3.5. Diagram to show how the two forms of abnormal chromosome 16 (α^+ and α^0) are arranged to give the different forms of α-thalassaemia.

to form tetramers of β ($\beta 4$) or haemoglobin H. Haemoglobin H is unstable and precipitates as the erythrocytes get older, forming rigid Heinz bodies which are removed during passage through the spleen. The damage to the membrane brought about by this removal results in a shortened red-cell life span. The Hb concentration is usually between 7 and 11 g/dl, the cells are hypochromic and show variation in size and shape. Both the MCV and MCH are reduced. Clinically, haemoglobin H disease is very variable. Some patients may be severely affected with a condition similar to the severe β-thalassaemias, while others are only mildly affected and live almost normal lives.

Deletion of 4 genes occurs in homozygous α^0-thalassaemia. No α-chains are formed and the predominant chain is γ, which forms tetramers ($\gamma 4$, haemoglobin Bart's). It does not function as an oxygen carrier but there is persistance in the fetus of the embryonic Hb Portland ($\zeta_2 \gamma_2$) which allows survival for a time, but death usually occurs between 25 and 40 weeks of gestation, or shortly after birth.

In summary, α-thalassaemia causes either stillbirth or, more usually, a mild disease with survival into adult life.

The α-thalassaemias are seen with greatest frequency in southeast Asia (Thailand, Malay peninsula and Indonesia), where haemoglobin Bart's is a frequent cause of stillbirths and haemoglobin H disease is common. They are also seen in the Mediterranean region and the Middle East, and a mild form also occurs in Africa. Sporadic cases have been reported in every racial group.

The β-thalassaemias

The β-thalassaemias result from a large number of abnormal genes, whose incidence and molecular characteristics vary between different races, and many are at present ill-defined. The most common abnormal genes are β^0 and β^+: in homozygotes, the β^0 chain results in no β chain production at all, whereas there is some chain production with the β^+ gene. The disorders produced by both chains are very similar and no distinction can be made on clinical grounds.

In no case has the precise molecular defect been identified; almost all the β-chain genes that have been examined have been found to be normal. On the other hand, there is a great deal of evidence that messenger RNA synthesis is abnormal. In some cases, no mRNA is produced at all, in others there is a reduced production, and in some, mRNA is transcribed but not translated into protein due to molecular defects, such as an inappropriately placed chain-termination codon.

β-thalassaemia has a world-wide distribution but is frequently seen in the Mediterranean region, parts of the Middle East, India, Pakistan and in south-east Asia. There is good evidence that its high incidence in these regions results from the gene bestowing a protective effect when heterozygous against *P. falciparum*.

Ever since the disease was described by Cooley in 1927, it has been clear that there is a very wide spectrum in its severity, ranging from people who have a normal haemoglobin concentration on one hand to still-birth on the other. The mild forms are termed thalassaemia minor and the severe forms thalassaemia major, but there is no clear-cut distinction between the two. Now that the genetic and laboratory aspects are clearer, it has been found that homozygotes usually have the major form and heterozygotes the minor form, but within each group there is a wide variability in the manifestation of the abnormal gene or genes and it is usually not possible to differentiate by clinical or laboratory tests those who are only moderately severely affected into homozygous or heterozygous categories without carrying out family studies. Improved laboratory diagnosis by electrophoresis of haemoglobin has also revealed that most β-thalassaemia heterozygotes are not anaemic at all.

The natural history of homozygous β-thalassaemia is that of a severe disease with patients rarely surviving into the third decade. The disease does not present at birth since production of fetal haemoglobin, $\alpha_2\gamma_2$, is not affected, but the infant becomes anaemic and jaundiced during the first few months of life, at the time when Hb A should be taking over from Hb F. The basic lesion is in the inability to produce β chains and hence there is an excess of α chains present in the red cell. The α chains precipitate within the cells and this leads to destruction of the red cells, mainly during the normoblastic stage in the marrow (ineffective erythropoiesis), but there is also a considerably shortened survival in the circulation as well. The response to the ineffective erythropoiesis is an enormous hypertrophy of the bone marrow with resulting skeletal changes which are a feature of the disease, mainly affecting the skull, long bones and hands. X-ray of the skull shows enlargement of the diploic spaces and radiating striations in the subperiostial bone, ('hair-on-end' appearance). These changes cause the typical 'thalassaemic' facies with bossing of the skull and enlargement of the upper maxillae producing prominent molar eminences and depression of the bridge of the nose. The long bones and hands show thinning of the cortex and osteoporosis, so that fractures are frequent and may be the presenting sign.

The excessive red-cell destruction (due to deposits of α-chain in the red cells) leads to considerable enlargement of the spleen, and this itself may lead to secondary hypersplenism with an increased rate of red cell destruction, combined with neutropenia and thrombocytopenia.

The profound anaemia (4–5 g/dl) has two other effects. First, there is a failure to grow, particularly striking in the case of muscle tissue, so that patients complain of weakness and low exercise tolerance, and have a characteristic stick-like appearance. Secondly, iron absorption from the gut is excessive, resulting in haemosiderosis, a major complication of thalassaemia major, from which the patients usually die before the age of 20 years. Iron deposition results in diffuse nodular cirrhosis of the liver, occasionally in diabetes mellitus, but most frequently of all in siderosis of the myocardium, with subsequent arrythmias and congestive cardiac failure. The iron deposition is probably also the cause of the failure to grow normally during puberty and the failure to develop secondary sexual characteristics.

The anaemia of thalassaemia is the result of ineffective erythropoiesis in the marrow combined with a shortened red-cell life span. The haematological changes in the peripheral blood are the formation of microcytic hypochromic red cells which also vary greatly in size and shape (Plate 1). The peripheral blood film is very similar to that seen in iron deficiency. In the latter case, however, the serum iron levels are always low, whereas in thalassaemia the iron concentration is high and the iron binding protein, transferrin, almost completely saturated with iron. Electrophoresis of haemoglobin from the homozygous patient shows the presence of Hb F and A_2, with a reduction or absence of Hb A, depending on whether the abnormal genes are β^0 or β^+.

Heterozygous β-thalassaemia shows a wide variation in severity. Most heterozygous patients are symptomless carriers usually unaware of any abnormality. Occasionally patients are found with moderate anaemia, leg ulcers and mild jaundice. Rarely, patients are as severely affected as in the homozygous form. In the symptomless carriers, the haemoglobin concentration is usually within normal limits, but the MCH may be low. The peripheral blood film usually shows a moderate degree of microcytosis with variation in size and shape and often the presence of target cells. The symptomless carriers may show a marked degree of anaemia during pregnancy and this may be associated with folate deficiency. Diagnosis is made by the electrophoresis of the haemoglobin, which usually shows an increase in Hb A_2. Hb F occasionally may be present in small amount (up to 7%). The thalassaemias are covered in detail in the monograph of Weatherall & Clegg (1981) and the short review of Modell (1976).

The disease is most commonly found in the areas delineated in Fig. 3.4.

Treatment. It is not possible to alter haemoglobin chain production at the present time and therapy centres around transfusion. There has been a big change in transfusion policy in the last few years: whereas patients were transfused previously when the haemo-globin values fell to 4–5 g/dl, they are now transfused approximately every 6 weeks with sufficient blood to keep them close to or within the normal range of haemoglobin concentration. This has had a profound effect on the children who now grow and mature normally and lead near normal lives (Modell 1976). If the spleen is considerably enlarged and there is clear evidence that it is also destroying the tranfused red cells and increasing transfusion requirements, then splenectomy is carried out. The main remaining complication is the haemosiderosis, aggravated by the transfusions, each unit of blood containing about 200 mg of iron. The patients thus still die in the second or third decade but the introduction of the iron-chelating agent, desferrioxamine, holds great promise for the future. This agent can be given subcutaneously overnight using a portable pump and it appears probable that the amount of iron excreted in the faeces and urine combined with the agent can at least be sufficient to prevent further iron accumulation (Bank 1978).

It is now possible to make an antenatal diagnosis of homozygous β-thalassaemia on blood obtained from a 20-week old fetus. The reticulocytes can be analysed for the presence or absence of β-chain production. Abortion is then carried out on those fetuses showing either no β-chain production (β^0-thalassaemia) or markedly reduced production (β^+-thalassaemia).

Haemolytic anaemias due to extrinsic causes

Haemolytic anaemias also result from causes primarily outside the red cell, that is, extrinsic causes. These are acquired diseases and there are a large number of different syndromes with which haemolytic anaemia is associated. The classification of Wintrobe (1967) takes up the whole of one page. Most of the syndromes are rare, but those most likely to be met with fall into the following 3 groups presented in order of their relative frequency. First, haemolysis secondary to other diseases such as leukaemia or reticulosis. Secondly, an idiopathic haemolytic anaemia unassociated with any other abnormality and thirdly, haemolysis brought about by drugs.

Secondary haemolytic anaemias

Haemolytic anaemia is found associated with leukaemia or with tumours of reticuloendothelial tissue or occasionally with infections, especially virus pneumonia. Haemolytic anaemia is often seen in lymphocytic leukaemia but rarely in myeloid leukaemia; it is also found in Hodgkin's disease, myelosclerosis, and is a well-recognized complication of reticulosarcoma, lymphosarcoma and giant follicle lymphoma. It is also seen in disseminated lupus erythematosus.

In most patients with this type of secondary haemolytic anaemia, the haemolysis is mild and is only a subsidiary feature of the disease; in a few patients, however, it may dominate the symptom-complex and in some it is the presenting symptom.

A small number of the patients in this group (possibly 10–20%) have antibody on their red cells and can thus be classified as the autoimmune type, as discussed in the next section.

Idiopathic autoimmune haemolytic anaemia
Patients with this disease are less common than those with haemolysis secondary to other disease. In the so-called idiopathic condition haemolysis dominates the clinical picture, but no evidence can be found of any other disease. The characteristic feature that is common to all these patients is that they have antibody on the surface of their red cells, which is almost certainly why the cells are destroyed prematurely. In most patients the nature of the antigen on the red cell with which the antibody reacts cannot be determined, but in a few patients the antibody reacts with some of the antigens of the Rh system.

The antibody found in these patients can be subdivided into two characteristic types, 'warm' antibody and 'cold' antibody (Dacie 1959). These terms refer to the fact that the antibody either reacts best with the red cell at 37°C (warm) or only at a temperature below 32°C (cold). As might be expected, the clinical picture is different in the two types.

When the warm antibody is present the disease is independent of external temperature and is found in both sexes and at all ages. It is very variable in its manifestation ranging from severe anaemia in acutely ill people to a mild chronic anaemia with few symptoms. Jaundice is common and splenomegaly is almost always found.

Patients who have cold antibody in their plasma present in an entirely different way and are said to be suffering from the cold agglutinin syndrome.

Since cold antibody only reacts with red cells at a temperature below about 32°C the symptomatology is dependent on external temperature, the condition being worse during the winter. Exposure to cold precipitates the appearance of Raynaud's phenomena, with cold, stiff, numb and purplish fingers. Toes, ear lobes and the nose may also be involved. These symptoms are due to the formation of agglutinates of red cells in the vessels of the skin as skin temperature frequently falls well below 32°C when exposed to the cold. Cold antibody attached to red cells also activates the complement system, and on rewarming, the red cells haemolyse, giving rise to haemoglobinaemia and haemoglobinuria.

The warm antibodies are non-agglutinating and must be demonstrated by the antiglobulin test (p. 134). The cold antibodies are agglutinators and can be demonstrated by the visible agglutination which occurs when the blood is cooled to room temperature.

Haemolytic anaemia due to drugs

The survival of red cells in the circulation for their normal life span of 120 days is dependent on the maintenance of the integrity of the structural component of the cell and also on the proper functioning of the various biochemical reactions. Any drug which affects essential structural components and functional activities is likely to bring about a shortening of red-cell life span, and it is not surprising, therefore, to find an increasing number of drugs which have been reported to cause a haemolytic process. When any haemolytic anaemia is encountered, it is necessary to enquire closely to determine whether there has been any exposure to drugs or chemicals (Dacie 1962; Worlledge, Hughes-Jones & Bain 1982).

The precise way in which many drugs act on the red cell is not known, but 3 categories of action can be recognized.

1   Certain chemicals, such as benzene, toluene and saponin, which are fat-solvents, may act on the red-cell membrane disrupting the lipid components.

2   Certain drugs, such as primaquine, sulphonamides, phenacetin, etc., act as oxidants resulting in a failure to maintain haemoglobin and other cell components in a reduced state. People with G6PD and other enzyme deficiencies are of course particularly sensitive to these drugs (p. 57), but if given in a large enough dose they will affect normal red cells.

3   Thirdly, there are drugs which will combine with components on the surface of the red cell and the resulting complex is antigenic. The antibody that is produced then reacts with the drug-

complex on the red-cell surface and brings about its destruction. Penicillin, when given in very large doses (more than 6 g/day), can occasionally bring about a haemolytic process in this way (White *et al*. 1968).

References

BANK A. (1978) The thalassaemia syndrome. *Blood*, **51**, 369.

BEUTLER E. (1959) The haemolytic effect of primaquine and related compounds: a review. *Blood*, **14**, 103.

COOLEY T. B. (1927) Von Jaksch's anemia. *Amer. J. Dis. Children*, **33**, 786.

DACIE J. V. (1959) Acquired haemolytic anaemias. *Brit. Med. Bull.*, **15**, 67.

DACIE J. V. (1962) Haemolytic reactions to drugs. *Proc. roy. Soc. Med.*, **55**, 28.

DACIE J. V. *The Haemolytic Anaemias* (2nd edn). Part I, 1960. Part II, 1962. Part III, 1967. Part IV, 1967. Churchill, London.

FRY J. (1961) Clinical patterns and course of anaemia in general practice. *Brit. med. J.*, **2**, 1732.

HADEN R. L. (1947) A new type of hereditary haemolytic jaundice without spherocytosis. *Am. J. Med. Sci.*, **214**, 255.

LEHMAN H. & HUNTSMAN R. G. (1974) *Man's Haemoglobins*. North Holland, Amsterdam.

MACKINNEY A. A. (1965) Hereditary spherocytosis. *Arch. int. Med.*, **116**, 257.

MODELL B. (1976) Management of thalassaemia major. *Brit. med. Bull.*, **32**, 270.

MOLLISON P. L. (1983) *Blood Transfusion in Clinical Medicine* (7th edn). Blackwell Scientific Publications, Oxford.

ROGERS D. W. & 5 others (1978) Early deaths in Jamaican children with sickle cell disease. *Brit. med. J.*, **1**, 1515.

WEATHERALL D. J. & CLEGG J. B. (1981) *The Thalassaemia Syndromes* (3rd edn). Blackwell Scientific Publications, Oxford.

WEATHERALL D. J. & CLEGG J. B. (1978) Molecular basis of thalassaemia. *Brit. J. Haemat.* suppl. to vol 31, 133.

WHITE J. M., BROWN D. L., HEPNER G. W. & WORLLEDGE S. M. (1968) Penicillin-induced haemolytic anaemia. *Brit. med. J.*, **3**, 26.

WINTROBE M. M. (1967) *Clinical Haematology*. Kimpton, London.

WORLLEDGE S., HUGHES-JONES N. C. & BAIN B. (1982) Immune haemolytic anaemias. In *Blood and its Disorder* (eds R. M. Hardisty & D. J. Weatherall), p. 479. Blackwell Scientific Publications, Oxford.

Recommended reading not mentioned in text

ALLGOOD J. W. & CHAPLIN H. (1967) Idiopathic acquired autoimmune haemolytic anaemia. A review of forty-seven cases treated from 1955 through 1965. *Am. J. Med.*, **43**, 254.

HUEHNS E. R. (1965) Thalassaemia. *Postgrad. med. J.*, **41**, 718.

HUTCHINSON H. E. (1967) *An Introduction to the Haemoglobinopathies*. Arnold, London.

EDITORIAL (1969) Glucose-6-phosphate dehydrogenase deficiency and favism. *Lancet*, **ii**, 1177.

Objectives in learning: haemolytic anaemias

1   To know the tests for recognizing (a) that an excessive rate of destruction of red cells is taking place and (b) that the marrow is producing cells at a rate in excess of normal.

2   To understand the principle involved in the division of haemolytic anaemias into intrinsic and extrinsic abnormalities and to classify aetiological factors in each division.

3   To understand the following aspects of hereditary spherocytosis: (a) mode of inheritance; (b) clinical features and modes of presentation; (c) laboratory findings specific for this disease.

4   To understand the role of glucose-6-phosphate dehydrogenase in the glycolytic cycle and the aetiology and clinical characteristics of the haemolytic anaemia which may be associated with a deficiency of this enzyme.

5   To understand the basic lesion of the haemoglobinopathies and the clinical and laboratory manifestations of sickle-cell anaemia and thalassaemia.

6   To understand the role of autoantibodies in the production of haemolytic anaemias and to know the types of disease with which they are associated.

PLATE LEGENDS

All the photographs of cells are of the same magnification. The preparations were stained with May–Grünwald–Giemsa stain.

Plate 1

(*a, top left*) *Normal*. Normal red cells are round, except where distorted by adjacent cells, and do not vary greatly in size They are well-filled with haemoglobin. Two platelets (darkly-stained) about 1–2 μm in diameter, are also shown.

(*b, top right*) *Hypochromic and microcytic cells*. Taken from a patient with iron-deficiency anaemia. Note the central pallor of the cells, the abnormal shapes and the considerable variation in size. Only some of the cells have diameters below the lower limit of normal.

(*c, lower left*) *Target cells*. Taken from a patient with thalassaemia major.

(*d, lower right*) *Macrocytes*. Taken from a patient with pernicious anaemia. Compare size with normal cells (*top left*).

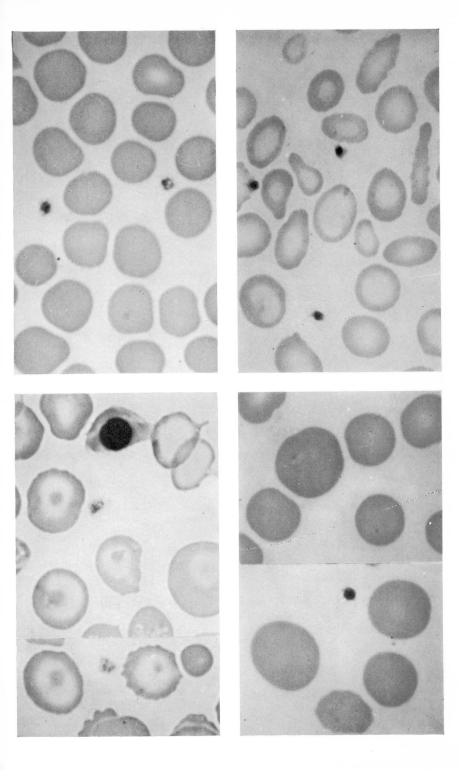

Plate 2

(*a, top left*). There is one spherocyte in the centre of each photograph. Taken from a patient with hereditary spherocytosis.

(b, top right) *Howell–Jolly bodies*. These are the single small round bodies in the red cells and are only seen in the absence of a functional spleen. Taken from a splenectomized patient with hereditary spherocytosis.

(*c, lower left*) Sickle cells. These cells were present in the peripheral blood film made soon after withdrawal of venous blood from a patient with sickle-cell anaemia (SS).

(*d, lower right*) *Abnormal haemoglobins*. Electrophoresis of haemoglobins on starch gel. The haemoglobins migrated from the left-hand side of the gel.
1   Normal haemoglobin A.
2   Patient with sickle cell trait; both haemoglobin A and S are present.
3   Patient with sickle cell anaemia; most of the haemoglobin is S, with a small proportion of haemoglobin F.
4   Patient with S and C haemoglobins. This results in a disease which is usually milder than in patients homozygous for S.

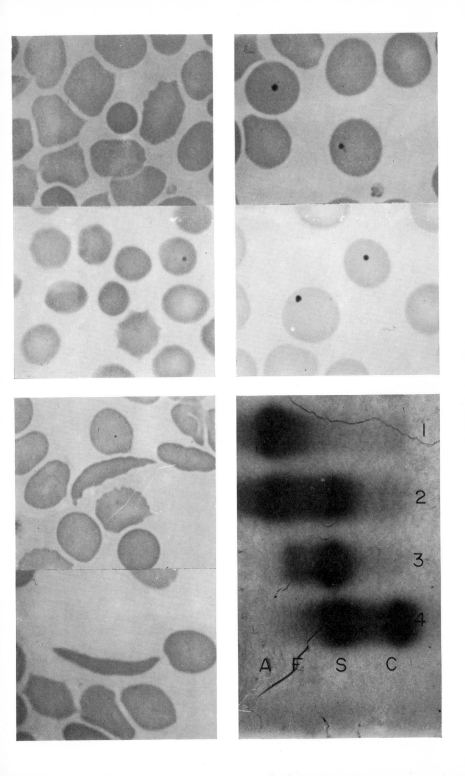

Plate 3

(*a, top left*) *Pronormoblasts*. An early stage in the maturation of red cells. Characterized by its large size and deep-blue staining of the cytoplasm.

(*b, top right*) *Normoblasts*. When this stage is reached in red-cell development, no further mitosis occurs. The lower two cells contain haemoglobin in the cytoplasm, which stains a blueish-red colour. Since the cytoplasm is blueish-red, the cell is termed a polychromatic normoblast. The nucleus is lost soon after this stage.

(*c, lower left*) *Reticulocytes*. The RNA that is present in red cells during the first 2 days in the peripheral blood is precipitated and stains blue with supra-vital dyes.

(*d, lower right*) *Megaloblasts*. These cells were present in a patient with pernicious anaemia. Identical changes are seen in folate deficiency. Note the larger size of the cell and the more delicate nuclear chromatin compared to the normoblast in the photograph above this one.

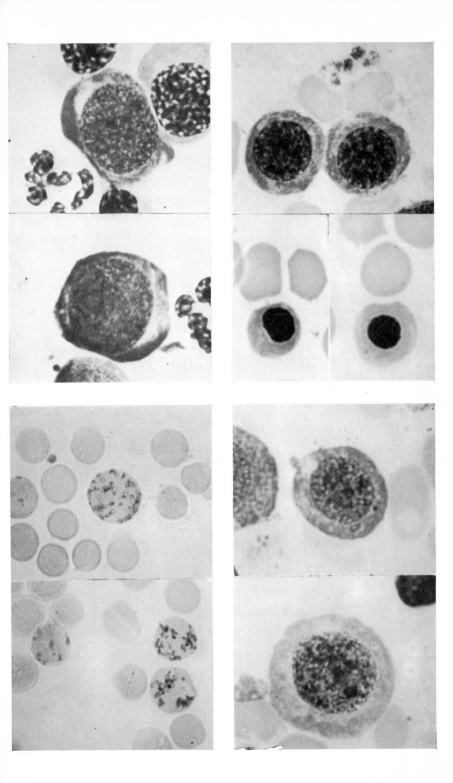

Plate 4

(*a, top left*) *Myeloblasts*. An early stage in the development of polymorphs. Note the nucleoli and absence of granules in the cytoplasm.

(*b, top right*) *Myelocytes*. A later stage in polymorph development. Note the granules in the cytoplasm and the absence of nucleoli.

(*c, lower left*) *Polymorphs*. Most polymorphs have less than 5 lobes under normal conditions.

(*d, lower right*) *Hypersegmented polymorphs*. Taken from a patient with pernicious anaemia. They are also seen in folate deficiency.

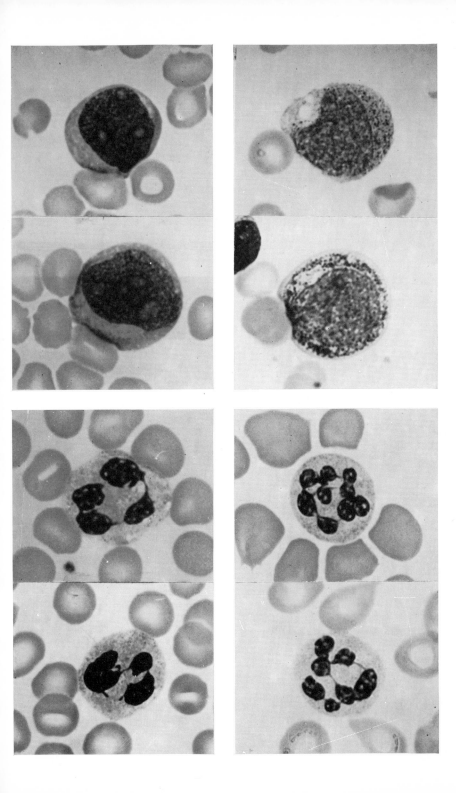

Plate 5

(*a, top left*) *Lymphoblasts*. Taken from the peripheral blood of a patient with acute lymphoblastic leukaemia.

(*b, top right*) *Lymphocytes*. These cells are only slightly larger than red cells and have only a small rim of cytoplasm.

(*c, lower left*) *Monocytes*. These large cells with irregularly-shaped nuclei are phagocytes. The vacuoles are probably due to the use of sequestrine as an anti-coagulant.

(*d, lower right*). *Infectious mononucleosis*. The increase in mononuclear cells in this condition is due to the presence of lymphocytes. Most of the cells are cytotoxic T cells produced in response to Epstein–Barr virus antigens present on the surface of B lymphocytes.

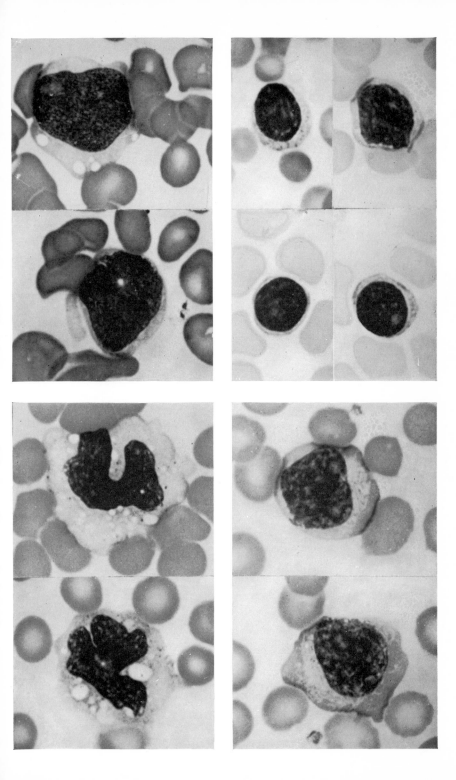

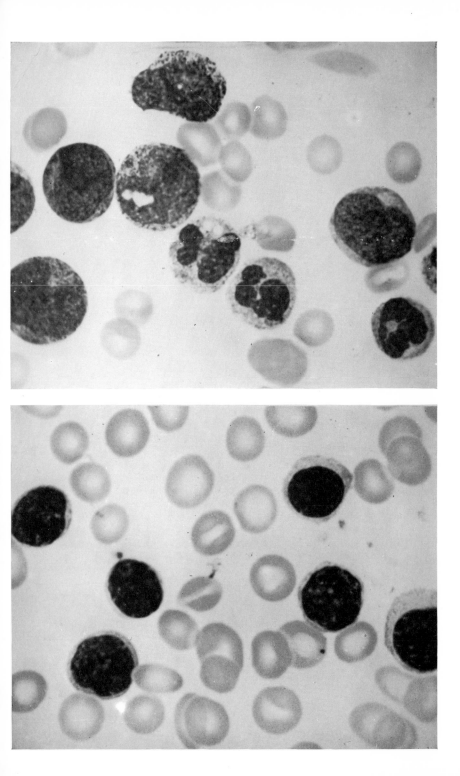

Plate 7

(*a*, *top left*) *Fetal red cells*. The darkly-staining cells are fetal red cells present in the maternal circulation. The maternal cells have lysed (acid-elution technique of Kleihauer).

(*b*, *top right*) *Heinz bodies*. These bodies represent denatured haemoglobin and are usually seen in patients who have glucose-6-phosphate dehydrogenase deficiency and who are either taking certain oxidant drugs or have ingested Fava beans. This photograph, however, is taken from a peripheral blood film of a patient with normal red-cell enzymes, but who had taken an excess of phenacetin. This drug overwhelmed the normal mechanisms for maintaining haemoglobin in the reduced state with the result that Heinz bodies were readily produced when the red cells were incubated with acetylphenylhydrazine. They are to be differentiated from Howell–Jolly bodies, which are nuclear remnants. Heinz bodies are demonstrated by staining with methyl violet.

(*c*, *lower left*) *Acute myelocytic leukaemia*. The predominant cell in the peripheral blood is the myeloblast.

(*d*, *lower right*) *LE cells*. This is a polymorph (note the typical darkly-staining multilobular nucleus squashed to one side of the cell) which has ingested a nucleus from another white blood cell. This phagocytic activity results from the presence of anti-nuclear antibody present in the patient's plasma.

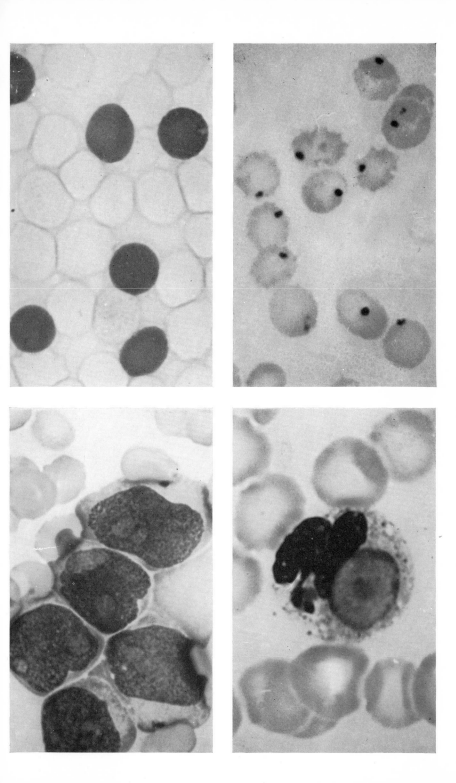

Plate 8

(*top*) *Megakaryocyte*. This is a very large cell found only in the bone-marrow; it is multinucleate and platelets bud from the periphery of the cytoplasm.

(*b, bottom*) Chromosome preparation by banding technique. Taken from a male with Ph[1]-positive chronic granulocytic leukaemia. A portion of the chromosome from the long arm of one of the No. 22 pair has been transferred to the long arm on one of the No. 9 pair (both positions arrowed). Reproduced with kind permission from The Chronic Leukaemias by D. A. G. Galton, in *Blood and its Disorders* (eds R. M. Hardisty & D. J. Weatheral), Blackwell Scientific Publications, Oxford (1983).

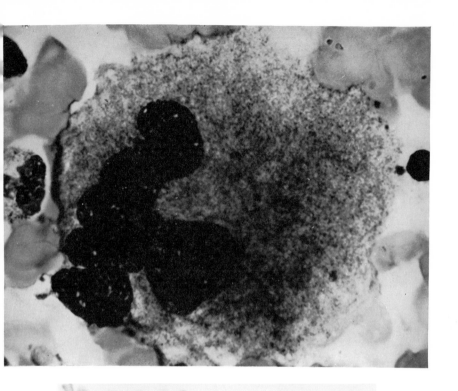

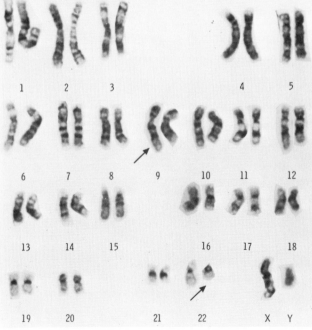

Chapter 4
Malignant and Non-Malignant Disorders of White Cells

The leukaemias

White cell development
All the formed elements of blood (red cells, neutrophils, monocytes, lymphocytes and platelets) are derived from a pluripotential stem cell mainly present in the bone-marrow, but also present in the spleen and peripheral blood. These pluripotent stem cells are self-renewing, but they also produce daughter cells, which become committed to one of the cell lines.

When a stem cell is committed to form lymphocytes, it divides within the bone-marrow and about 80% of the small lymphocytes seen on bone marrow biopsy are newly-formed cells. The cells (both T and B cells) then pass to the peripheral blood to continuously recirculate between the lymph nodes, lymph and back to the blood. The life span of lymphocytes is still conjectural. If unstimulated by antigen, they may only survive for a few weeks. If the B cells are stimulated and proceed as far as plasma cells, they produce a great deal of antibody but can no longer divide and are thus also short-lived.

In the adult, the myeloid series also arises only in the bone marrow and proceeds through the myeloblast and myelocyte stages into mature polymorphs (Plate 4a,b,c) and the whole process takes approximately 12 days. Once in the peripheral blood, polymorphs have an average life span of only about 10 hours, and they do not return to the circulation once they have left it.

Classification
Leukaemia can be looked upon as a neoplastic process involving the precursors of the white cells of the blood. There is an abnormal proliferation of cells of either the myeloid or of the lymphocyte series. There are four common varieties of leukaemia: acute lymphoblastic, acute myeloid, chronic granulocytic and chronic lymphocytic. The term chronic myeloid leukaemia is sometimes used

73

synonymously with chronic granulocytic leukaemia but it is preferable to use chronic myeloid leukaemia as a generic term for five separate diseases of which the Philadelphia-chromosome-positive granulocytic leukaemia is by far the commonest. The other four are rare and will not be considered here.

The classification of leukaemia into one of these types is important because therapy depends on classification. The most marked clinical difference is between the acute form of the disease of either cell type on the one hand and the chronic forms of either cell type on the other.

Aetiology

The aetiology of leukaemia is still an enigma, although it is known that it can result from ionizing radiation, from toxic chemicals, such as benzene, from exposure to certain myelo-toxic drugs and from virus infection. The evidence for ionizing radiation is based on finding an increased incidence under the following circumstances: in the survivors of the nuclear bomb explosions at Hiroshima and Nagasaki; in patients with ankylosing spondylitis treated with irradiation; in children born to mothers who have been submitted to diagnostic radiology; and in radiologists. Radiation induces acute and chronic myeloid and acute lymphoblastic leukaemia but not chronic lymphocytic. Court-Brown & Doll (1959) observed that there was an increasing incidence of both acute and chronic myeloid leukaemia in Britain between 1945 and 1957 and suggested that this was the result of an increasing exposure to ionizing radiation in medical diagnosis. However, figures from the U.S. published in 1967 (Franmeni & Miller 1967) show the first recorded decrease in mortality from leukaemia and it is suggested that this is the result of the more conservative use of X-rays and the wider use of radiological devices that greatly reduce radiation exposure. Studies made at Hiroshima indicated that the threshold for induction of leukaemia was about 20 rads, whereas in the case of children who had been subjected to pre-diagnostic irradiation, the threshold was as low as 200 mrads.

Recently, a retrovirus (human T cell leukaemia/lymphoma virus, or HTLV) has been isolated from patients presenting with adult T-cell leukaemia/lymphoma. This adult T-cell leukaemia is endemic in a localized area in Japan, but clusters and isolated cases have been found elsewhere.

Epidemiology

The age incidence of the different forms of leukaemia show distinctive differences. Chronic lymphocytic leukaemia is the only one which resembles most neoplasms in that it shows a progressive increase from the age of about 40 years onwards. The myeloid leukaemias, both acute and chronic, show two components; namely, a plateau between 30 and 40 years and a peak at about 70–80 years. Acute lymphoblastic leukaemia on the other hand has its highest incidence before 20 years.

Clinical picture

Signs and symptoms common to all leukaemias

All the leukaemias share signs and symptoms in common arising from the infiltration by neoplastic cells of bone marrow, spleen, lymph nodes, liver and other organs such as the brain, although the extent of organ involvement varies with both the types of disease and the stage of development. The infiltration of bone marrow with leukaemic cells replaces the normal tissue and results in decreased red cell production, neutropenia and thrombocytopenia. The commonest findings are thus anaemia, infections and abnormal bleeding (chiefly purpura, epistaxis, bleeding from the gums and bruising).

Infections may be due to bacteria, fungi or viruses, either as local lesions, e.g. around the mouth, or as pneumonia or septicaemia. The organisms are usually the common ones, such as *Staph. aureus*, *Pseudomonas aeruginosa* and *Klebsiella*, although they may be of the opportunistic category. The basal metabolic rate is sometimes raised, resulting in excessive sweating and loss of weight.

Both the acute and chronic forms may show signs and symptoms resulting from infiltration of the skin, nervous system or bone (causing bone pains and a limp in children). Furthermore, haemorrhage may occur into the nervous system, eye or internal ear. Although these features are common to all the leukaemias, there is a marked difference between the acute and chronic leukaemias in their mode of presentation.

Acute leukaemias. The acute form is characterized by the finding of a severely ill patient with symptoms present for only a few days or weeks. The commonest findings are anaemia, fever and abnormal bleeding. There may be some enlargement of the liver, spleen and lymph nodes, although these findings are usually absent in adults, especially during the early phase of the disease.

Remission of the disease may rarely occur spontaneously but more often follows treatment, and may last a few weeks or months. In the case of acute lymphoblastic leukaemia in children, there may be a permanent cure.

Chronic leukaemias. The presentation of the chronic form of the disease is, on the other hand, quite different, and it is not uncommon for the disease to be discovered accidentally while carrying out a peripheral blood examination for some unrelated reason. Initially, the patients are only mildly ill and give a history of symptoms that have been present for several months. The commonest presenting symptoms are loss of energy, tiredness and shortness of breath. A less common complaint is of abdominal enlargement due to splenomegaly. In contrast to the acute leukaemias, enlargement of the liver and spleen is commonly present and may be gross; in chronic lymphocytic leukaemia, the lymph nodes are usually enlarged. However, it is not always possible to distinguish with any certainty between the lymphocytic and myeloid types on clinical grounds; lymph nodes are often enlarged in the more active stages of chronic myeloid leukaemia, and are not always present in lymphocytic leukaemia.

A haemolytic process is present in a minority of patients with chronic lymphocytic leukaemia, varying in intensity from a mild to a predominating and severe process, and is usually associated with a positive direct antiglobulin test.

In the chronic lymphocytic variety, apart from the abnormal growth of the lymphocytes, there is also a functional failure of immune mechanisms. This results in a reduction of immunoglobulin levels in the plasma and in the reduced ability to make antibodies. About two-thirds of patients with chronic lymphocytic leukaemia have immunoglobulin levels below normal, and the greater the reduction, the more frequently infection is found. The neutropenia which is so frequently found also predisposes to infection.

Peripheral blood and bone-marrow biopsy

Morphology in the acute leukaemias
In the peripheral blood in acute lymphocytic leukaemia, most of the nucleated cells are lymphoblasts and lymphocytes; in many

instances the blasts are small but can usually be distinguished from normal mature lymphocytes, whereas in other cases, the blasts are larger with more cytoplasm. There are usually one or two nucleoli. The bone-marrow is usually cellular; most of the cells are lymphocytes, as in the peripheral blood.

In acute myeloid leukaemia there may be greater variety of cell types with both blood and marrow showing similar patterns. In some cases, almost all the cells may be blasts, but in others, more mature forms such as promyelocytes and myelocytes may be present. Myeloblasts usually have more nucleoli than lymphoblasts and are larger with more cytoplasm.

In a small minority of patients, differentiation of myeloblasts from lymphoblasts is difficult based on morphology alone and more sophisticated cytochemical tests are needed. Positive reactions for peroxidase and with Sudan Black characterize myeloblasts whereas the presence of aggregates of glycogen staining with periodic-acid-Schiff are characteristic of lymphoblasts.

It is characteristic of both forms of acute leukaemia that there is a reduction, often marked, of the mature segmented polymorph.

Morphology of the chronic leukaemias
In the chronic leukaemias, cells more mature than blasts predominate in the peripheral blood.

In chronic granulocytic leukaemia, myelocytes and polymorphs predominate over blasts, in contrast to the acute form of the disease where blast cells predominate. The myelocyte (Plates 4b and 6a) is a cell which is as large as, or larger than, a myeloblast but which is distinguished from it by the absence of nucleoli and the presence of granules in the cytoplasm. Some nuclei show an indentation; this is the first stage in the development of the nucleus into the multilobular form. Almost all patients also have an increase in both basophils and eosinophils.

Three other features are frequently found in chronic granulocytic leukaemia. First, there may be an alteration in the number of platelets. Thrombocytosis is usual, the platelet count increasing up to values of $400-1000 \times 10^9$/litre (normal range $150-400 \times 10^9$/litre); less commonly, there is a thrombocytopenia. Secondly, there is an increase in vitamin B_{12} concentration, due to the fact that leucocytes normally produce a protein carrier of B_{12} and this protein is produced in excess. Thirdly, the neutrophil alkaline phosphatase is low in about 90% of patients and is a useful diagnostic feature.

In chronic lymphocytic leukaemia the predominant cell is the mature lymphocyte (Plate 6b). Intermediate cells between the early lymphoblast and the mature lymphocyte are uncommon and are difficult to recognize with certainty.

White cell count in all types of leukaemia

The number of white cells in the peripheral blood is usually increased, but this is not an essential feature of leukaemia. About one-third of patients with acute leukaemia have white-cell counts within or even below the normal range ($4-10 \times 10^9/l$) during some stage of the disease, and the remainder have white-cell counts which usually fall in the range $10-50 \times 10^9/l$. In chronic forms of the disease, the white-cell count is elevated, usually to between $50 \times 10^9/l$ and $500 \times 10^9/l$.

There is a characteristic change in the leucocyte count with time in chronic granulocytic leukaemia. The number of cells increases with time and the rate of increase is found to be exponential; that is, the number doubles at regular intervals, the actual interval in which doubling takes place varies between patients, and is often over 70 days (Fig. 4.1). The increase in total leucocyte count is accompanied by an increase in the size of the spleen and by a fall in haemoglobin concentration.

Sequence of changes in chronic granulocytic leukaemia

The survivors of the atomic bombs in Japan in 1945 have been intensively studied, with the result that the progression of changes in chronic granulocytic leukaemia have been elucidated (Kamada & Uchino 1978). The appearance of the Ph^1 chromosome (see p. 80) is probably the first manifestation of the disease and it was calculated that if all the leukaemic cells were derived from a single cell with a Ph^1 chromosome, then it would take about 6 years for the leucocyte count to reach about $100 \times 10^9/l$. The earliest change in the peripheral blood is the raising of the leucocyte count above the upper limit of normal ($10 \times 10^9/l$) due to the presence of leukaemic cells. At the same time, basophilia, thrombocytosis and the low leucocyte alkaline phosphatase make their appearance. As the count rises to $20,000 \times 10^9/l$, the percentage of myeloblasts and myelocytes in the peripheral blood rises above 5% of the total white-cell count and the increase in serum vitamin B_{12} becomes apparent. Splenomegaly is found when the count is in the region of $50,000 \times 10^9/l$ and shortly after that symptoms arise.

All patients with chronic granulocytic leukaemia develop a more rapidly progressive terminal phase, although the exact form which this takes shows considerable variation between patients. In general, there is an increase in malaise and in wasting, with night sweats, bone pain, infection and haemorrhage accompanied by a fall in haemoglobin concentration and platelet numbers and a rise in white-cell count, with a predominance of the more immature blast cells.

Progression of changes in chronic lymphocytic leukaemia

Dameshek (1967) considered chronic lymphocytic leukaemia to be a gradual accumulation of inactive but long-lived lymphocytes. Progression should therefore be stepwise and with this basis in mind, Rai *et al.* (1975) analysed 125 patients and found that four stages in the disease can be characterized, each progressive stage being associated with a shorter life span (Table 4.1). Thus, at stage 0 there was only lymphocytosis ($> 15 \times 10^9/l$) and more than 40% of bone marrow cells were lymphocytes; this stage was associated with an average survival of some 10–20 years from the time the stage was diagnosed, the longest lived patient being still alive after 32 years. In stage I, the lymph nodes became palpable and the average survival from then onward was 8 years. Stage II was characterized by lymphocytosis with enlargement of the liver or spleen or both, and the average survival was 6 years. Stage III was characterized by lymphocytosis and anaemia (haemoglobin

Table 4.1. Characteristic features for the staging of chronic lymphocytic leukaemia. The sign ⊞, gives the essential feature indicating the stage reached

Stage	Lympho-cytosis blood & marrow	Lymph nodes	Spleen & liver	Anaemia	Thrombo-cytopenia
0	⊞	—	—	—	—
I	⊞	⊞	—	—	—
II	⊞	+ or −	⊞	—	—
III	⊞	+ or −	+ or −	⊞	—
IV	⊞	+or −	+ or −	+ or −	⊞
Average life span (years)	10–20	8	6	1–2	1–2

concentration, < 11 g/dl) and the average survival was 1–2 years. In the final stage, IV, lymphocytosis and thrombocytopenia were present (platelet count, $< 100 \times 10^9/l$) and the average survival time still shorter. These stages should prove to be a useful guide to prognosis.

Bone-marrow biopsy

The diagnosis of leukaemia must be substantiated by an examination of haemopoetic tissue in the bone-marrow. One of the main purposes of this examination is to exclude the presence of other diseases, e.g. secondary carcinomatous deposits, myelosclerosis and multiple myeloma, which also result in immature white cells being found in the peripheral blood. In leukaemia there is a great increase in the number of white-cell precursors relative to the red-cell series. In the acute leukaemias, the predominating cells are either myeloblasts or lymphoblasts. In chronic granulocytic leukaemia, the predominating cell is the myelocyte and in chronic lymphocytic leukaemia, there is heavy infiltration with lymphocytes. There is usually a decrease in the total number of cells of both the red-cell series and megakaryocytes, which parallels the anaemia and thrombocytopenia.

An interesting feature of the leukaemias is the finding of chromosome abnormalities in the white cells. The discovery in 1956 that man had 46 chromosomes and the techniques that led to this observation stimulated chromosome studies in leukaemia. The principle finding is the presence of the Philadelphia chromosome (Ph[1]) in chronic granulocytic leukaemia and many will not make the diagnosis unless it is present. It is not unique to chronic granulocytic leukaemia, occasionally being found in the acute leukaemias. In about 90% of Ph[1]-chromosome-positive patients, there is a translocation of material from the long arm of chromosome 22 to the long arm of chromosome 9; in the remainder, the translocation occurs to other chromosomes. What is left of chromosome 22 is called the Philadelphia chromosome (it was first observed in that city). It appears to be the Ph[1] chromosome which is intimately associated with the pathogenesis of the disease.

Abnormalities are commonly seen in the acute leukaemias, but there are great variations from patient to patient and no characteristic karyotype is associated with a particular disease. About half the patients have no detectable abnormalities. When an abnormality is present there may be loss or duplication of chromosomes or translocation may occur. There is much discussion as to whether the chromosome abnormalities are causal or consequential and the problem is unresolved. The abnormalities can occasionally be of help in the diagnosis of atypical cases.

Treatment

Leukaemia is usually an incurable disease (except for acute lymphoblastic leukaemia in children); in the case of the chronic leukaemias, treatment may prolong life for up to 1 year or possibly more. The main object of treatment is the improvement in wellbeing of the patient. In many cases almost normal health can be restored and patients may continue to work until within a few weeks of death. As in the other forms of neoplastic disease, specific treatment aims at the suppression of cell division, and this can be brought about by ionizing radiations or by drugs. The type of treatment is different for the three diagnostic categories: chronic granulocytic leukaemia, chronic lymphocytic leukaemia and acute leukaemia.

Chronic granulocytic leukaemia

In this form of the disease the treatment is aimed at reducing the leucocyte count to normal limits, as experience has shown that this is followed by a marked alleviation of symptoms and rise in haemoglobin concentration. Reduction in leucocyte count can usually be brought about by treatment with the alkylating agent, busulphan (myeleran) which is a powerful suppressant of cell division, or by intermittent radiotherapy to the spleen. Busulphan is administered until the leucocyte count falls to almost normal limits. If the busulphan is then stopped, the leucocyte count will start to rise again within a few days, and usually at a faster rate than before therapy was started. If the doubling time of the leucocyte count is over 70 days (i.e. relatively slow) then busulphan can be given intermittently, but if it is faster than this, a continuous maintenance dose is given. An example of the effect of treatment on the leucocyte count and haemoglobin concentration is given in Fig. 4.1, taken from the excellent review of Galton (1959) on the treatment of chronic leukaemias. A trial (Medical Research Council 1968) has shown that busulphan therapy is superior to radiotherapy in the treatment of chronic myeloid leukaemia.

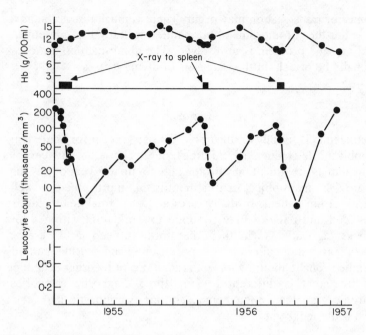

Fig. 4.1. The changes in haemoglobin concentration and leucocyte count in a patient with chronic myelocytic leukaemia following X-ray therapy to the spleen. Note the increasing rate of rise of leucocyte count after the second and third courses of treatment. Redrawn from Galton (1959).

Chronic lymphocytic leukaemia

In contrast to chronic granulocytic leukaemia there is no definite relationship between the total lymphocyte count and the severity of the symptoms. The patients mainly complain of symptoms due to the large size of the spleen or lymph glands, or of symptoms due to anaemia, infection, or haemorrhage resulting from thrombocytopenia. Treatment is aimed at improving anaemia and thrombocytopenia and at controlling the symptoms. It is doubtful whether symptomless patients should be treated at all. If the enlargement of the spleen and lymph nodes causes symptoms, these organs can be reduced in size by radiotherapy and by the alkylating agent, chlorambucil.

Anaemia, neutropenia and thrombocytopenia may respond to chlorambucil or to corticosteroids. The bone-marrow in lymphocytic leukaemia is very susceptible to ionizing radiation and alkylating agents, and a hypoplastic condition can easily be produced. This danger has to be weighed against possible benefits of treatment.

Acute leukaemias

The treatment of choice in acute leukaemia is chemotherapy and stems from the observation that folate antagonists (methotrexate) would induce a remission. The many chemical agents now available fall into 4 groups. First, the *anthracycline antibiotics* (daunorubicin); these intercalate with DNA base pairs and inhibit DNA synthesis. Secondly, *alkylating agents* (busulphan, chlorambucil); these are activated with the appearance of highly reactive groups which disrupt DNA. Thirdly, purine and pyrimidine analogues (thioguanine, mercaptopurine, cytosine arabinoside); these become incorporated into DNA and block transcription. Fourthly, vincristine and vinblastine; these block microtubule polymerization in the formation of mitotic spindles and thus inhibit mitosis. These agents are usually given in combination and dosage schedules are continuously being revised, based on empirical observations of their relative efficacy. Acute lymphoblastic leukaemia of childhood is the disease which most readily responds and an initial remission rate of over 90% can now be achieved by a combination of prednisone and vincristine with or without other drugs; if a remission is achieved prophylactic irradiation of the central nervous system is carried out and therapy continued for a further 2·5 years with two anti-mitotic agents. Many relapse, but about one-third attain long-term, disease-free survival.

Acute myeloblastic leukaemia is more difficult to treat. A remission is only achieved if a dose of drugs is given which is sufficient to produce marrow hypoplasia for several weeks. This requires intense supportive therapy for the anaemia, neutropenia and thrombocytopenia. Complete remission has been reported to be achieved in 25–70% of cases, but relapse usually occurs after an average of 6–12 months, although a small number have been kept disease-free for many years.

Bone-marrow transplants, both allogeneic and autologous, have been used for AML with some success. The main advantage is that treatment of the patient prior to transplantation can be much more effective. The problems are: failure to engraft; rejection; recurrence of leukaemia and graft-versus-host disease. The hope for the future lies in autologous grafts with removal of leukaemic cells *in vitro* before return to the patient.

Leukaemoid reactions

Occasionally patients are seen in whom the peripheral blood findings suggest at first sight that they could have leukaemia, but in reality the changes are an unusual response to some other disorder. The blood picture may resemble that seen in chronic granulocytic leukaemia or that of chronic lymphocytic leukaemia. Leukaemoid reactions resembling acute leukaemia are rare.

In the myelocytic type, an arbitrary definition of a leukaemoid reaction is the finding of a total white-cell count of over $50 \times 10^9/l$ and the presence of immature white cells (myeloblasts and myelocytes) in the peripheral blood. This abnormal reaction sometimes occurs as the result of infection, especially in children, and also in patients with malignant tumours. When compared with chronic granulocytic leukaemia, the percentage of immature cells in the peripheral blood is usually much lower in the leukaemoid picture, the anaemia is slight or absent, the number of platelets is usually normal (although thrombocytosis may occur) and the alkaline phosphatase in the polymorphs is normal or increased (not reduced as in chronic granulocytic leukaemia).

The leucoerythroblastic anaemias may also require to be differentiated from the true leukaemic process. The former occur as the result of bone-marrow infiltration, usually by secondary deposits of carcinoma, but is also seen in myelosclerosis and multiple myeloma. The characteristic feature is the presence of an anaemia with an increase in the number of nucleated red cells (normablasts) and also the presence of a few immature white cells, usually myelocytes, but without much increase in the white-cell count.

Lymphocytic leukaemoid reactions may be seen as an excessive response to infection, usually infectious mononucleosis and pertussis.

A bone-marrow aspiration may be necessary for the differential diagnosis; it may reveal either bone-marrow infiltration (carcinoma, fibrosis, myeloma) or, in the case of leukaemoid reactions secondary to infection, show only minor changes in morphology, compared to the far more intense myelocytic or lymphocytic infiltration seen in leukaemia.

Infectious mononucleosis (glandular fever)

This is generally a benign infectious disease caused by the Epstein–Barr virus, with an incubation period of about 5–7 weeks. The virus can be found in saliva, and transmission is by droplets or by kissing. Most of those infected have very mild or subclinical attacks and infection is clearly widespread as about 90% of adults are found to have EBV-related antibodies. The most common symptoms and signs are malaise, fever and sore throat. It is almost impossible to distinguish on clinical grounds the pharyngitis of infectious mononucleosis from that due to other viral or bacterial infections. The posterior cervical lymph nodes are almost invariably enlarged and, in a minority of patients, there is widespread lymphadenopathy. In about half the cases, there is a moderate splenomegaly. Very occasionally there may be thrombocytopenic purpura, haemolytic anaemia, hepatitis, myocarditis or central nervous system involvement (Banatvala 1970). Further details on the clinical aspects can be obtained from the review of Pullen (1973).

The two characteristic findings in the peripheral blood are an absolute increase in the number of lymphocytes above the upper limit of normal of $3 \cdot 5 \times 10^9/l$, usually up to values of $10–20 \times 10^9/l$ and the appearance of lymphocytes with abnormal morphology (Plate 5d). The morphological appearances are variable and difficult to describe and the recognition of the cells depends on experience with microscopical techniques. The morphology has been reviewed by Carter (1966). The atypical lymphocytes are mainly T cells, but there is also an increase in the number of B cells. The B cells are infected with virus (only B cells have a receptor for EBV) and the T cells represent a cellular response to the B cells which have virus-encoded antigens on their surface.

In about 80–90% of patients, heterophile antibodies which react with sheep red cells (Paul–Bunnell reaction) develop during the second and third weeks of the illness and then decline and are usually undetectable after 2–3 months. Hetrophile antibodies are those which cross-react with antigens of the cells of other animal species; that is, they react with an antigen different from that which initiated the immune response. Antibodies against proteins produced by the virus also appear at the same time and then persist for years, giving lasting immunity.

References

BANATVALA J. E. (1970) Infectious mononucleosis. Recent developments. (Annotation.) *Brit. J. Haemat.*, **19**, 129.

CARTER R. L. (1966) Review of some recent observations on 'glandular fever cells'. *J. Clin. Path.*, **19**, 448.

COURT-BROWN W. M. & DOLL R. (1959) Adult leukaemia. Trends in mortality in relation to aetiology. *Brit. med. J.*, **1**, 1063.

DAMESHEK W. (1967) Chronic lymphocytic leukaemia – an accumulative disease of immunologically incompetent lymphocytes. *Blood*, **29**, 566.

FRANMENI F. & MILLER R. W. (1967) Leukaemia mortality. Downturn in the United States. *Science*, **155**, 1126.

GALTON D. A. G. (1959) Treatment of chronic leukaemias. *Brit. Med. Bull*, **15**, 78.

KAMADA N. & UCHINO H. (1978) Chronological sequence of appearance of clinical and laboratory findings characteristic of chronic myelocytic leukaemia. *Blood*, **51**, 843.

MEDICAL RESEARCH COUNCIL (1968) Chronic granulocytic leukaemia. Comparison of radiotherapy and busulphan therapy. Report of MRC working party for therapeutic trials in leukaemia. *Brit. med. J.*, **1**, 201.

PULLEN H. (1973) Infectious mononucleosis. *Brit. med. J.*, **2**, 350.

RAI K. R., SAWITSKY A., CRONKITE E. P., CHANANA A. D., LEVY R. N. & PASTERNAK B. S. (1975) Clinical staging of chronic lymphocytic leukaemia. *Blood*, **46**, 219.

Recommended reading not mentioned in text.

HOUGIE C. (1965) Early diagnosis and natural history of chronic lymphatic leukaemia. *Ann. Int. Med.*, **45**, 39.

ROSENTHAL N. (1935) Leukaemia. Its diagnosis and treatment. *J. Amer. med. Ass.*, **104**, 702.

Objectives in learning: leukaemia

1   To understand the basis for the differentiation of leukaemia into acute and chronic forms based on the clinical picture and on the peripheral blood findings.

2   To know the characteristic morphology of the white cells in the peripheral blood in the common types of leukaemia—chronic myeloid and lymphocytic leukaemia, and the acute leukaemias.

3   To know the characteristic changes with time in the white-cell count in chronic myeloid leukaemia, and the relationship between the white cell count and the clinical symptoms.

4   To know the cause of the symptoms in chronic lymphocytic leukaemia.

5   To know the basic principles (but not the details) of treatment in (i) acute leukaemia; (ii) chronic myeloid leukaemia, and (iii) chronic lymphocytic leukaemia.

Chapter 5
Aplastic Anaemia, Agranulocytosis, Polycythaemia Vera, Myelosclerosis and Drug Reactions

Aplastic anaemia is a syndrome in which there is a failure of cell production and it is characterized by a pancytopenia, i.e. a reduction in the number of red cells, neutrophils and platelets in the peripheral blood; there is also a decrease in the amount of haemopoietic tissue in the bone marrow. No other evidence of a disease process, such as leukaemia or carcinomatous deposits, can be detected. It is an uncommon syndrome, the incidence in Europe being about 1–3/100,000 and there are almost certainly a number of aetiological factors producing the same clinical picture.

The first description of the disease was made by Ehrlich in 1888. In his patient a pancytopenia was present and this was accompanied by an acellular bone marrow. Although a hypocellular marrow due to a considerable decrease in the amount of haemopoietic tissue is the normal finding on bone-marrow biopsy, this is not always the case; occasionally a normal or even hypercellular biopsy is obtained. The most likely explanation in many cases is that there are local foci of haemopoietic activity in a marrow which is in general hypoplastic and a larger specimen of marrow obtained by iliac crest trephine may give a better picture of bone marrow activity.

Although red cells, leucocytes and platelets are usually all reduced in number, there is considerable variation between patients in that one of the cellular elements may be reduced to a much greater extent than the others. A reticulocytopenia is an important feature in diagnosis and in severe cases with a poor prognosis, the reticulocytes may be $<10 \times 10^9$/l, neutrophils $<0.5 \times 10^9$/l and platelets $<20 \times 10^9$/l, combined with a hypocellular marrow ($<20\%$ haemopoietic tissue). The symptoms are those of anaemia combined with infection, often fulminating due to the absence of polymorphs. Haemorrhage into the skin, or from the gastrointestinal, genital or urinary tracts, or haemorrhage into the brain results from the thrombocytopenia. The clinical course is variable. In some there is a rapid progression to death within

3–6 months, while a few may remit, if they can be kept alive with transfusions of red cells and platelets and the use of antibiotics during the aplastic phase. If the patient survives for a year, there is then a good chance of complete recovery.

As far as aetiology is concerned, about half the cases in Europe occur in an older age group, many of whom have been on anti-rheumatic drugs such as the pyrazolones (phenylbutazone) or propionic acid derivatives (buprofen). Chloramphenicol and gold are also common agents, but there is a long list of drugs including antibiotics, anticonvulsants, antithyroid and antihistamines which have been incriminated. Benzene is the only common industrial chemical which regularly produces aplastic anaemia if given in sufficient dose; paints, glues and other industrial solvents can also do so. Possibly about one-third of all cases are thought to be due to drugs or chemicals.

In children and young adults, aplastic anaemia may develop about 10 weeks after a hepatitis A or non-A, non-B infection and has a very poor prognosis.

Treatment of aplastic anaemia requires regular blood transfusions and a proportion of patients may show a significant response to androgens. Bone-marrow transplantation is indicated for severe aplastic anaemia, if a suitable compatible donor is available.

Agranulocytosis

The term agranulocytosis refers to a disease characterized by an acute illness with necrotizing lesions of the mouth and throat associated with very few or a complete absence of polymorphs in the peripheral blood. It is a rare condition and in about one-third to half the cases, it is possible to attribute the disease to the side-effects of certain drugs. The platelets and red cells are not affected. The first drug to be incriminated was amidopyrine, and although this compound is no longer prescribed, it is still available in some proprietary preparations in certain parts of the world. The incidence of agranulocytosis in those taking the drug has been reported to be as high as 1%. Many other drugs will cause agranulocytosis, some of the most common being: antithyroid drugs, especially thiouracil (1–2% of those taking the drug); the tranquillizers such as chlorpromazine; some sulphonamides and chloramphenicol. Many of these drugs also cause aplastic anaemia. The known mechanism of action of these drugs is either through an antigen–antibody reaction or through suppression of DNA synthesis (p. 94).

The disease should always be suspected in a patient presenting with a severe infection of the throat and sometimes elsewhere, accompanied by profound weakness and exhaustion, especially if the patient is known to be taking any drug. The treatment is withdrawal of any suspected drug and the use of antibiotics. The mortality rate is high; Israëls (1962) states that the prognosis is better if there are some white-cell precursors in the marrow than when these are absent.

Polycythaemia rubra vera

Polycythaemia rubra vera (also known as primary proliferative polycythaemia) is a disease in which there is an uncontrolled proliferation of red cells, neutrophils and platelets. The aetiology is similar to chronic granulocytic anaemia in that the neoplastic cells are derived from a single clone. This has been shown by finding that in women with polycythaemia vera, all the neoplastic cells contain the same polymorphic variant of the X-linked glucose-6-phosphate dehydrogenase, whereas the non-neoplastic cells contain either one or the other. Polycythaemia vera is generally considered to be a relatively benign type of neoplasm giving rise to a chronic disease from which the patient ultimately dies. It is to be distinguished from polycythaemia secondary to anoxia due to living at high altitudes, or secondary to respiratory or cardiac disease. It is also well established that polycythaemia can occur secondary to cerebellar haemangioblastomas, renal tumour and uterine fibroids. It is thought that there is excessive erythropoietin production in these latter diseases.

Recently, it has become evident that heavy smoking can also cause polycythaemia, sometimes accompanied by a leucocytosis. The total red cell mass is above normal and falls to normal limits on stopping smoking. It is not due to lowering of pO_2 levels but may be due to a stimulatory component in tobacco smoke (Sagone & Balzercak 1975). Occasionally, patients are found in whom examination of the peripheral blood shows a haemoglobin concentration and PCV just above the normal range but who do not have an increased total red cell volume, as measured by ^{51}Cr-labelled red cells. The apparent polycythaemia in these people is due to a reduction in plasma volume.

Although the term polycythaemia indicates an increase in the number of red cells, the diagnosis is based on an increase in haemoglobin concentration and PCV as well as the red-cell count. The haemoglobin concentration in untreated patients is above 17 g/dl in women and 18 g/dl in men, and the PCV is in the range 0·55–0·8. If there is any doubt about whether polycythaemia exists or not the red-cell volume should be estimated with ^{51}Cr-labelled red cells (Mollison 1983). In polycythaemia vera, the total red-cell mass is in excess of the normal range of 27–33 ml/kg. Estimation of red-cell volume does not differentiate between polycythaemia vera and polycythaemia secondary to anoxaemia, as there are similar increases in volume in both.

In polycythaemia vera, a small increase in the total leucocyte count is seen in about 70% of patients (Calabresi & Meyer 1959) and white-cell counts are usually between 10 and 30 × 10^9/l at the time of diagnosis. The increased rate of production of the white-cell series in the marrow is frequently reflected by the finding of a few immature white cells (myelocytes) in the peripheral blood. Most patients have a rise in platelet count (400–2000 × 10^9/l) associated with an alteration in morphology (variation in size and shape) and in function. The total volume of haemopoietic tissue in the marrow is increased at the expense of fatty tissue and this is best shown in a section taken from a trephine biopsy. A bone-marrow biopsy should always be carried out to exclude the presence of any other disease.

If the patient survives 5–25 years and does not die from a thrombosis or haemorrhage, the blood and clinical pictures may slowly change. In some patients (10–20%) the signs of myelofibrosis appear, that is, the replacement of the marrow by fibrous tissue, and there is a great increase in the size of the spleen, which contains haemopoietic tissue. Other patients, perhaps 10%, develop acute myeloid leukaemia as a terminal event. The numbers of patients developing these changes is increasing, but it is not clear whether this is part of the natural history of the disease which is showing up because the length of life has been greatly prolonged by ^{32}P therapy, or whether the ^{32}P therapy itself is inducing a leukaemic change.

An integral and important part of the disease is the development of vascular thrombosis and haemorrhage. In Videbaek's series from Copenhagen (1950), nearly one-third of the patients had thrombotic episodes and these accounted for 20% of the deaths.

The thromboses are mainly cerebral, cardiac or mesenteric. The incidence of vascular occlusion has been found to be correlated with the PCV. Pearson & Wetherley-Mein (1978) found the higher the PCV, the greater the number of occlusive episodes. Patients with a PCV value of over 0·6 have occlusive episodes at a rate of almost 1 each year (Fig. 5.1). These results also show that the PCV should be kept below 0·45 by treatment in order to avoid such episodes.

About 10% of patients have peptic ulcers, an incidence higher than in the normal population, and this is thought to be due to thrombosis of smaller vessels. The thrombosis is probably due in part to the slowing of the circulation in the peripheral vessels due to increased viscosity of the blood, and in part to the raised concentration of platelets.

Haemorrhage is also an extremely important complication, Videbaek (1950); finding it in 50% of his cases, and it was the cause of death in 30%. Haemorrhage is a common complication of surgery. The cause of the bleeding is not well-understood. The platelets are found to be large and have an abnormal shape and there are also functional changes as shown by the diminished response to aggregating agents such as ADP (see p. 98).

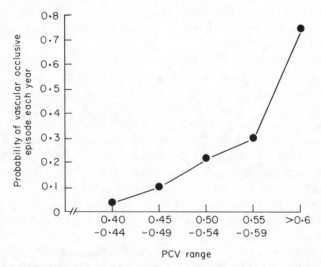

Fig. 5.1. The probability of the occurrence of a vascular occlusive episode related to the PCV. A probability of 0·1 indicates a 1 in 10 chance of the occurrence. Adapted from Pearson & Wetherley-Mein (1978).

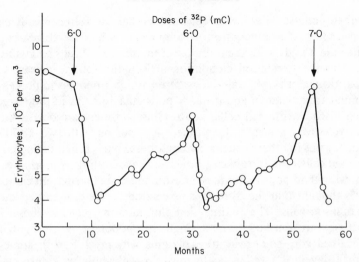

Fig. 5.2. The effect of giving three doses of ^{32}P on the erythrocyte count of a patient with polycythaemia vera. Adapted from Szur, Lewis & Goulden (1959).

In the early stages of the disease there may be no symptoms and a raised haemoglobin concentration may be an incidental finding. When red-cell volume is increased, the patient presents with a florid dusky-red cyanotic colour of the face, lips, hands and feet. Generalized pruritis, especially on exposure to heat, is a common symptom. Apart from the skin manifestations, the only other abnormality is an enlarged spleen in most patients.

Venesection is an important way of relieving symptoms and is the method of choice in the first instance. If this does not achieve control, then patients may be treated by chemotherapy (bulsuphan is the most widely used reagent) but many haematologists believe that the most successful treatment is irradiation of the bone-marrow using intravenous radioactive phosphorus (^{32}P) (Szur *et al.* 1959). Several courses may be required. Successful therapy reduces the incidence of thrombotic and haemorrhagic episodes, and the average length of life from diagnosis in a recent series has been 13 years, compared to 6 years without ^{32}P treatment (Fig. 5.2).

Myelofibrosis

Myelofibrosis is an uncommon disease in which the haemopoietic tissue of the bone-marrow is slowly replaced by fibrous tissue and sometimes also by bony trabeculae. It is characterized clinically by the finding of a large spleen together with a leucoerythroblastic anaemia, that is, with the presence of immature red cells and white cells in the peripheral circulation. The nature of the disease is unknown, but is generally considered to be a neoplastic process similar to leukaemia and primary polycythaemia. As in the latter two diseases, the red cells, neutrophils and megakaryocytes are derived from a single clone since in a person with two G6PD isoenzymes in other tissues only one isoenzyme is found in haemopoietic cells. The fibroblasts, however, have both the isoenzymes, showing that they are not derived from the same pluripotent clone. It is thought that the fibrosis is a reaction to the presence of the neoplastic cells. The finding that the abnormal cells in these 3 diseases are derived from a single haemopoietic pluripotential stem cell goes some way to explaining why myelofibrosis sometimes develops into an acute myeloid leukaemia as a terminal phase and similarly polycythaemia vera and chronic granulocytic leukaemia can develop a myelofibrotic phase. The diagnosis is made by performing a bone-marrow trephine and demonstrating replacement of haemopoietic tissue by reticulin, collagen fibres, and fibroblasts.

Drug reactions

The effect of drugs on the formed elements of blood has been discussed in several chapters but is briefly summarized again here in order to get an overall picture of drug reactions as far as the haematological system is concerned.

Drug reactions manifest themselves in four different ways. There may be an effect on the precursors of all the formed elements resulting in marrow aplasia and pancytopenia (p. 80), or red cells, polymorphs and platelets may be affected separately, manifesting as a haemolytic anaemia (p. 70), agranulocytosis (p. 89) or thrombocytopenic purpura (p. 105). Whenever any of these conditions are found in patients it is extremely important to determine whether drugs could play any part in the aetiology, since the only hope of cure is removal of the drug.

Certain drugs are used as myelosuppressive agents, such as busulphan and chlorambucil, and these need not be discussed further. The drugs that are of greater concern are those which have a deleterious action on the haematological system as a side-effect to the purpose for which they are primarily given. During the last few decades, three of the mechanisms of these side-effect activities have been established, although much remains to be discovered.

1   There are those drugs which are oxidants and which bring about oxidation of many substances in the red cell including the compounds NADH, NADPH, reduced glutathione and haemoglobin. These drugs will regularly cause a haemolytic anaemia if given in large enough doses, but the patients who are especially sensitive are those who have G6PD deficiency (p. 57). Examples of these drugs which react in this way are primaquine, some sulphonamides and phenacetin.

2   Other drugs act through an antigen–antibody reaction. These drugs combine with surface constituents on red cells, polymorphs or platelets and this may result in the formation of antibody acting specifically against the drug attached to the surface of the formed element. The presence of antibody on the surface of the formed elements leads to their premature destruction. Examples of the drugs which act in this way are: for red cells, penicillin; for polymorphs, amidopyrine, some sulphonamides, and thiouracil; for platelets, quinine, quinidine, some sulphonamides, and sedormid.

3   Chloropromazine has been found to suppress DNA synthesis in white-cell precursors in the marrow and thus brings about agranulocytosis. Chloramphenicol inhibits protein synthesis by mitochondria.

4   In *chronic lead poisoning*, the lead brings about mitochondrial and ribosomal abnormalities and inhibits several enzymes concerned with haem synthesis. The result is an anaemia with a small reduction in mean cell haemoglobin concentration. There is agglutination of the ribosomes which are still present within reticulocytes, and in films of peripheral blood stained with May–Grünwald–Giemsa these agglutinates appear as the characteristic punctate basophilia (small, round, blue particles) whereas in normal cells, the ribosomes give rise to a diffuse blue-red staining (the polychromatic cell, p. 162).

The condition is most frequently seen in young children and is usually the result of chewing or biting objects coated with lead paint. The clinical syndrome is frequently associated with pica and is characterized by pallor, abdominal pain and constipation; irritability occurs later and eventually leads to coma and convulsions.

It can be seen that some drugs act through more than one

mechanism. Only a few of the commoner drugs which affect the formed elements of blood have been mentioned, but there are a greater number of other drugs which are known to be harmful, although for many drugs only one or two instances have been described. As new drugs are produced, so the list of those which affect red cells, polymorphs and platelets is extended. The incidence of drug reactions is in most cases extremely low so that, except in the case of amidopyrine, the benefits of most drugs far outweigh the deleterious effect seen in a few people.

References

CALABRESI P. & MEYER O. O. (1959) Polycythaemia vera. I. Clinical and laboratory manifestations. *Ann. Int. Med.*, **50**, 1182.

EHRLICH P. (1888) Uber einen Fall von Anämie mir Bermerkungen über regenerative Veranderunges des Knochenmarks. *Charité-Annalen*, **13**, 300.

HAVARD C. W. H. & SCOTT R. B. (1963) Refractory anaemia. A disease or a syndrome. *Lancet*, **i**, 461.

ISRAËLS M. C. G. (1962) Drug agranulocytosis and marrow aplasia. *Proc. roy. Soc. Med.*, **55**, 36.

MOLLISON P. L. (1983) *Blood Transfusion in Clinical Medicine* (7th edn). Blackwell Scientific Publications, Oxford.

PEARSON T. C. & WETHERLEY-MEIN G. (1978) Vascular occlusive episodes and venous hematocrit in primary proliferative polycythaemia. *Lancet*, **ii**, 1219.

SAGONE A. L. & BALZERCAK S. P. (1975) Smoking as a cause of erythrocytosis. *Ann. int. Med.*, **82**, 512.

SZUR, L., LEWIS S. M. & GOULDEN A. W. G. (1959) Polycythaemia vera and its treatment with radioactive phosphorus. *Quart. J. Med.*, **28**, 397.

VIDEBAEK A. (1950) Polycythaemia vera. Course and prognosis. *Acta med. Scand.*, **138**, 179.

Recommended reading not mentioned in text

DACIE J. V. (1982) Haemolytic reaction to drugs. *Proc. roy. Soc. Med.*, **55**, 28.

BARRETT K. E. (1970) Polycythaemia. *Practitioner*, **204**, 780.

Objectives in learning: effect of drugs

To know the mechanism of action and clinical manifestations of drugs disturbing both the normal development of haemopoietic tissue and the physiology of the red cells, polymorphs and platelets in the peripheral blood.

Chapter 6
Haemostasis and Abnormal Bleeding

The cessation of bleeding following trauma to blood vessels results from three processes: (i) the contraction of vessel walls; (ii) the formation of a platelet plug at the site of the break in the vessel wall; (iii) the formation of a fibrin clot. The clot forms within and around the platelet aggregates to form a firm haemostatic plug. The relative importance of these three processes probably varies according to the size of the vessels involved. Thus, in bleeding from a minor wound, the formation of a haemostatic plug is probably sufficient in itself, whereas in larger vessels, contraction of the vessel walls also plays a part in haemostasis. The initial plug is formed almost entirely of platelets but this is too friable on its own and must be stabilized by fibrin formation.

Although the action of platelets, the clotting mechanism and the integrity of the vascular wall are all closely related in the prevention of bleeding, it is convenient in the diagnosis of abnormal bleeding to attempt to classify the abnormality into one of these three systems. The commonest cause of bleeding is undoubtedly that resulting from a deficiency of platelets; the second commonest cause is an abnormality in the clotting mechanism. The remaining patients do not have any demonstrable lesion of platelets or clotting mechanism and hence they are placed in the group of vascular abnormalities, but there is no satisfactory test which is specific for vascular abnormalities. As new factors in the platelets and the clotting mechanism come to light, some of the so-called vascular defects will no doubt be reclassified within the other two systems.

A clinical distinction can frequently be made between bleeding due to clotting defects and bleeding due to a diminished number of platelets. Patients with clotting defects usually present with abnormal bleeding into deep tissues, muscles or joints. On the other hand, patients with a deficiency of platelets usually present with superficial bleeding, purpura, bruising and bleeding from epithelium, as from the nose or uterus. A further useful clinical distinction is that bleeding usually persists from the time of injury in the case of platelet deficiency, since platelet numbers are inadequate to form a good platelet plug, whereas in clotting defects, the initial bleeding may cease in the normal time since platelet plugs are readily formed, but the failure to form an adequate clot means that the platelet plug is not stabilized by fibrin formation and subsequently disintegrates and prolonged bleeding ensues. The clinical distinction is by no means complete, as deep-seated haemorrhage is sometimes found in platelet deficiency and, on the other hand, superficial bleeding and purpura occur in clotting defects.

It is convenient to consider platelet deficiency and clotting abnormalities separately.

Platelets

Platelet physiology

The blood platelets are formed in the bone-marrow by the fragmentation of the cytoplasm of the megakaryocytes. They are small (2–4 μm in diameter, Plate 1) and are normally present in a concentration of 150×10^9 to $400 \times 10^9/l$ of whole blood. Following their release from the marrow, their life span is of the order of 10 days. This has been determined by labelling platelets with radioactive chromium (^{51}Cr). The shape of the survival curve obtained from radioactively labelled platelets is neither linear nor exponential and is difficult to interpret: it has been suggested that the platelets are delivered to the circulation with a potential life span of about 10 days, but that there is also some random destruction irrespective of their age (Fig. 6.1). The sites of normal platelet destruction are not known.

The main function of the platelets is the formation of the haemostatic plug, which incorporates several different physiological mechanisms (Mustard & Packham 1977). First, there is the adherent property of platelets which enables them to stick to collagen, basement membrane and subendothelial fibrils. Within 1–2 seconds after the platelets have become attached to exposed subendothelial structures, they change their shape from a disc to a more rounded form and release the content of their granules, the most important substance being adenosine diphosphate (ADP). The platelets are also stimulated to produce prostaglandins (especially thromboxane A_2). These two compounds, ADP and thromboxane A_2, then cause other platelets to become attached at the

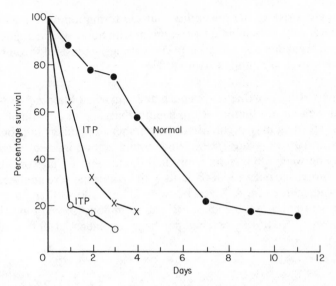

Fig. 6.1. Platelet survival curves: (●), normal survival; (×), mild idiopathic thrombocytopenic purpura; (○), severe thrombocytopenic purpura. Adapted from Barkham, P. (1966) *Brit. J. Haemat.*, **12**, 25.

site of the lesion to form aggregates, which are built up to form the platelet plug. The three processes (adherence, release of granules and aggregation) are known to be separate processes as certain rare bleeding disorders have been found to be due to platelet abnormalities involving only one of these three stages.

When platelets aggregate, they promote clotting in two ways. First, they are able to initiate contact activation of factor XII (p. 110) of the intrinsic pathway. Secondly, they are able to absorb other clotting factors to their surface and this considerably enhances the speed of the clotting reaction. Factors VIII and IX are adsorbed and potentiate factor Xa formation and then factors Xa and V are adsorbed and this results in a 1000-fold increase in the rate of conversion of prothrombin to thrombin (factor IIa). Platelets are also responsible for the contraction of the fibrin clot once it has been formed. Thus, the surface of a platelet is a site where fibrin formation can take place, leading to the development of the fully stabilized haemostatic plug.

A significant point concerning the ADP mechanism of adherence is that it can be inhibited by breakdown products of ADP and this gives rise to the possibility that the formation of thombi can theoretically be inhibited by treatment with non-toxic analogues of these breakdown products, especially if the synthesis of thromboxane A_2 is also inhibited with aspirin.

Petechial haemorrhages, purpura and abnormal bleeding

It is well known that petechial haemorrhages, purpura and abnormal bleeding may occur when the number of platelets falls below $100 \times 10^9/l$. Gaydos *et al.* (1962) found a good inverse relationship between the platelet count and the number of days on which haemorrhage occurred if patients with leukaemia were analysed as a group (Fig. 6.2). At levels between 20 and $100 \times 10^9/l$, purpura, bruises and nose bleeds were the commonest symptoms, but below $20 \times 10^9/l$, gross haemorrhage (melaena, haematemesis,

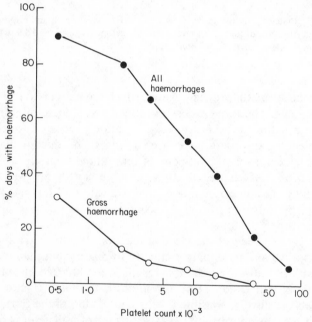

Fig. 6.2. Relationship between the platelet count and the number of days, expressed as a percentage, on which haemorrhage occurred in 92 patients with leukaemia: (●) all haemorrhages include petechiae, ecchymoses, epistaxis, haematuria, melaena and haematemesis. Note that the gross haemorrhage only occurred when the platelet count fell below 20,000/mm³. Adapted from Gaydos *et al.* (1962).

haematuria) become increasingly common. However, there is a great deal of variation in the relationship between the platelet count and haemorrhage in individual patients. Other factors clearly play a part in the control of haemostasis.

The reason for the occurrence of spontaneous haemorrhage when the platelet count is low is not known, but two possible mechanisms can be suggested. One, that the minor trauma associated with normal movement of the body causes capillary damage and that there is an insufficient number of platelets to form an adequate plug to prevent bleeding. The other suggested mechanism is that platelets continuously play a normal role in strengthening capillary walls by becoming attached and continuously incorporated into capillary endothelium. Although there is some evidence for the latter suggestion it is by no means substantiated.

Purpura is the collective term for bleeding into the skin or mucous membranes. The small haemorrhages up to pin head size are petechiae and larger haemorrhages are ecchymoses. The problem posed to the physician by a patient with purpura is a complex one, since the bleeding is the end result of an abnormality in haemostasis which may result from a variety of causes, and purpura may be found associated with a large number of disease conditions. The solution of the problem must therefore be attempted in two stages.

1 Determination of the nature of the abnormality in the physiological process that results in bleeding; i.e. whether the defect is due to a low platelet count, a functional abnormality of the platelets, or a deficiency of a clotting factor.
2 Correlation of this abnormality with others that may be present in order to obtain a diagnosis of the disease process (e.g. failure of platelet production by megakaryocytes due to marrow infiltration by leukaemic tissue).

Patients presenting with purpura as a main sign can be separated into those with low platelet counts (thrombocytopenic) and those with normal platelet counts (non-thrombocytopenic). The non-thrombocytopenic group can be subdivided into those rare patients who have qualitative platelet defects and the larger group who have vascular abnormalities. The latter is a miscellaneous group and contains such diseases as purpura senilis and purpura of infectious diseases and will not be discussed further.

Division into the thrombocytopenic and non-thrombocytopenic

groups can be carried out by estimating the number of platelets in the peripheral blood. Patients with bleeding manifestations resulting from a deficiency of platelets have a platelet count of below $100 \times 10^9/l$. If the patient is found to have a low platelet count, the next procedure is to determine whether this is due to the failure of platelet production by the megakaryocytes or whether it is due to a shortened life span of the platelets. The presence or absence of megakaryocytes in the bone-marrow must be determined by sternal marrow biopsy.

Failure of platelet production. If megakaryocytes are few or absent, it may be assumed that platelet production is at fault. The bone-marrow biopsy may also reveal other features which indicate the nature of the disease if evidence has not already been obtained from the peripheral blood. Thus, there may be a generalized failure of the bone-marrow (aplastic anaemia) which is either of unknown aetiology, or may be due to drugs or chemicals. Another cause of a reduced platelet production from megakaryocytes is displacement by leukaemic cells, lymphoma, reticulo-sarcoma and secondary carcinoma.

Shortened platelet survival. If the megakaryocytes in the marrow are numerous, then the thrombocytopenia is usually due to an excessive rate of removal of platelets from the peripheral circulation. In most cases the destruction results from antibodies attached to the platelet surface and the disease is termed autoimmune thrombocytopenic purpura.

Occasionally purpura due to destruction of platelets by mechanical means may be seen as an incidental finding in diseases dominated by other symptomatology. For instance, platelets can be destroyed by trapping in a large spleen (hypersplenism), by trapping in the vessels of a cavernous haemangioma, by destruction following adsorption of viruses and bacteria to their surface, or they may be damaged by the structural changes seen in small blood vessels in renal disease (microangiopathic thrombocytopenia).

The bleeding time and capillary resistance tests. The bleeding time test was introduced in 1910 by Duke, not as a diagnostic procedure, but as a means of following the progress of patients with thrombocytopenic purpura. When carried out under standardized conditions, it still remains the best clinical screening test that we have for the estimation of platelet function.

The most sensitive method of estimating the bleeding time is by making a small wound in the skin of the forearm after applying a blood-pressure cuff to the upper arm and inflating to 40 mmHg; the time that elapses until bleeding ceases is then measured (method of Ivy). The normal range is usually stated to be 2–8 minutes. Details of several methods of carrying out the test are well discussed by Abildgaard *et al.* (1968) and by Mielke *et al.* (1969). Since the wound only damages small vessels, haemostasis is mainly dependent on the formation of a platelet plug and hence the bleeding time is prolonged when platelet numbers are reduced. It is almost always normal in the presence of clotting defects.

The bleeding time is dependent on both the number of platelets in the plasma and on the extent of their functional activity. When the functional activity is normal, then there is a good correlation between the platelet count and the bleeding time measured in minutes (Harker & Slichter 1972) (Fig. 6.3). Bleeding times are not prolonged until the platelet count has fallen to $100 \times 10^9/l$. Below that value, there is a progressive and proportional prolongation in bleeding time, the time lengthening from the normal average of about 4·5 minutes to reach about 30 minutes as the platelet count falls to $10 \times 10^9/l$. Below $10 \times 10^9/l$, bleeding times may be prolonged to 1 hour or more.

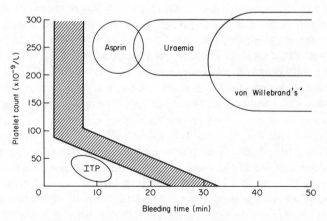

Fig. 6.3. The relationship between the platelet count and the bleeding time. The hatched area gives the relationship for platelets with normal functional activity. In autoimmune thrombocytopenic purpura (ITP), the platelets are younger and functionally more efficient. In uraemia, von Willebrand's disease and after taking aspirin, there is a functional impairment of platelet activity.

On the other hand, when there are functional changes in platelet activity, bleeding times are either shorter or longer than might be expected from platelet numbers. For instance, in the autoimmune thrombocytopenias, almost all the platelets are younger than normal and are functionally more efficient. The bleeding times are thus shorter than might have been expected from platelet numbers (Fig. 6.3). In contrast, there is a functional impairment of platelet activity in uraemia and in von Willebrand's disease and after the ingestion of aspirin, resulting in bleeding times that are prolonged despite platelet numbers in the normal range (Fig. 6.3). Aspirin has a moderate effect on the bleeding time and values usually fall between 8 and 20 minutes after a 300–600 mg dose. This prolongation is sufficient to provoke abnormal bleeding in certain people and aspirin is contraindicated in those with bleeding disorders. Aspirin acts by acetylating cyclo-oxygenase and thus inhibits thromboxane synthesis with a subsequent reduction in platelet aggregation. The effect of a single dose of aspirin can be detected for 1 week, i.e. until most of the platelets present at the time of taking the aspirin have been replaced by those newly synthesized.

, The bleeding time is thus most useful when there are moderate to gross changes in functional activity of the platelets and, when combined with an estimate of platelet numbers, can differentiate between decreased and increased function.

The capillary resistance test (Hess's test) is carried out by determining the number of petechiae developing in the antecubital fossa on application of a blood-pressure cuff to the upper arm, inflated to 80 mmHg. There are two reasons why this fails to provide useful diagnostic information concerning bleeding disorders. First, it is a non-specific test and is not only positive in certain disorders of haemostasis, but is also positive in a number of other diseases, such as various infectious diseases, scurvy, and chronic renal disease; it is also positive in a small number of apparently healthy individuals. The phenomenon of the development of petechiae on the application of a tourniquet was first described in 'hospital fevers' in 1810 and a century later it was described in association with scarlet fever, as well as with thrombocytopenic purpuras. Hess's original paper (1914) described the use of the test in patients with scurvy. Secondly, it is not a reliable screening test for bleeding disorders. It is very variable in its results, as different numbers of petechiae are found in the same person at different times and it is not always positive in the presence of thrombocytopenia. If a bleeding disorder is present in a patient, estimation of platelet numbers, bleeding time and coagulation tests will have to be carried out, whether the capillary resistance is positive or negative.

Idiopathic autoimmune thrombocytopenic purpura

The occurrence of a disease which is characterized by purpura, bruising and spontaneous bleeding from mucous membranes was first described by Werlhof in 1735. The association of these characteristics with a deficiency of platelets was recognized nearly 100 years ago. No other abnormality or causative factor could be found and hence the disease was termed idiopathic. During 1949–54, Ackroyd showed that thrombocytopenia in patients taking the sedative sedormid is due to the formation of an antibody against a complex of sedormid and the platelet; his explanation of the phenomenon is that sedormid forms a very labile union with the surface of the platelet and that the antibody then combines with the sedormid–platelet complex and this leads to the destruction of the platelets (Ackroyd 1962). These findings led others to search for anti-platelet antibodies in idiopathic thrombocytopenia. There is now substantial indirect evidence that many but not all patients with a clinical diagnosis of idiopathic thrombocytopenic purpura have autoantibodies in their plasma directed against their own platelets which results in a shortened life span due to premature platelet destruction in the spleen. The original evidence for the existence of antibodies was obtained *in vivo* by Harrington *et al.* (1951) who showed that sera taken from these patients and injected into normal people would cause prolonged thrombocytopenia (Fig. 6.4). The causative factor in the plasma was later shown to be an IgG immunoglobulin. This explanation is also consistent with the observation that children born to mothers with thrombocytopenic purpura also have thrombocytopenia for the first few days of life, as would be expected since IgG antibodies are known to cross the placenta.

The platelet life span has been shown to be shortened in all patients with immune thrombocytopenic purpura. The measurement of life span has been carried out by labelling with radioactive ^{51}Cr and is often reduced to about 1–2 days or less compared to the normal life span of 10 days. Surface counting over the spleen and liver has shown that in approximately 30% of patients the

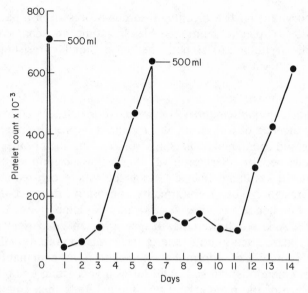

Fig. 6.4. The effect on the platelet count of a normal person who received two tranfusions of 500 ml of plasma from a patient with idiopathic thrombocytopenic purpura. The reduction in platelet count was due to the presence of anti-platelet antibodies in the donor's plasma. Redrawn from Harrington (1951).

destruction takes place only in the spleen, but in the rest the liver plays a part in destruction.

Clinical features. Autoimmune thrombocytopenic purpura presents in both an acute and chronic form. The acute form is seen at all ages but is most common before the age of 10 years, and two-thirds of patients give a history of a viral infection (upper respiratory tract, rubella) preceding the purpura by a few days to 2–3 weeks. Platelet counts are usually less than $10 \times 10^9/l$. The disease in most patients runs a self-limiting course of 1 week to 6 months but approximately 20% proceed to the chronic form, that is, lasting more than 6 months. The disease is almost always self-limiting when there is a history of preceding infection. The mortality is low, the main danger being intracranial bleeding.

The chronic form occurs mainly in the age period 10–30 years although it is sometimes seen in older subjects; it has a higher incidence in women than in men. The chronic form is usually not severe and mortality is low; platelet counts are usually between 20 and $80 \times 10^9/l$. Spontaneous cures are rare and the disease is characterized by relapses and remissions.

In a large series described by Doan *et al.* (1960) about one-third of the patients had petechiae and ecchymoses as the only presenting signs. The remainder also had bleeding from the following sources in order of frequency: nose, gums, vagina, gastrointestinal and renal tract. Cerebral vascular bleeding occurred in 3%. As a general rule the spleen is not palpable; when it is palpable it usually, but not always, rules out the diagnosis.

In order to make a diagnosis, bone-marrow biopsy must be carried out. In idiopathic thrombocytopenia, megakaryocytes are increased in numbers (up to four- to eightfold) and in size. An absence of megakaryocytes rules out the idiopathic disease. The marrow biopsy also serves the purpose of determining the presence of any other abnormality, such as aplastic anaemia, leukaemia or marrow infiltration by other forms of malignant tissue. Thrombocytopenia is sometimes the first symptom of systemic lupus erythematosus so that a search for LE cells must also be made. Thrombocytopenia due to drugs must also be excluded (p. 94).

Treatment. In the acute form of the disease, over 80% recover whatever the form of treatment. Corticosteroids have been widely used, but there is evidence that they have no effect on the duration of thrombocytopenia, and in one study appeared to defer recovery (Lusher & Zeulzer 1966). Nor is there any evidence that it decreases the number of patients who proceed to the chronic form (Schulman 1964). On the other hand, steroids are very useful in the chronic forms of the disease, about 70–90% having a partial remission. Splenectomy should be considered if the disease persists after 1–2 years and about two-thirds of the patients will respond to the treatment, some permanently, but some will relapse again after an interval.

It is possible to make an assessment of the effect of splenectomy by determining the site of sequestration of ^{51}Cr-labelled platelets; splenectomy carried out when there was only splenic sequestration resulted in remission in 90% of patients, but was a failure in 70% of patients when hepatic sequestration also took place (Najean & Ardaillon 1971). It should be stressed, however, that others have found a good response to splenectomy even when destruction is mainly hepatic (Aster 1972). Azothioprine can be used in a final attempt to reduce antibody formation and has been reported to be successful.

Platelet transfusions

It is often possible to raise the platelet count temporarily by platelet transfusions. The main indication for platelet transfusion is severe haemorrhage due to thrombocytopenia when the cause is diminished platelet production. When thrombocytopenia results from excess destruction, as in the presence of platelet antibodies, the response to transfusion is poor. Transfusion may also be indicated in a patient with thrombocytopenia prior to surgery. The platelets are transfused as platelet concentrations and should be given within 24–72 hours of withdrawal from the donor. Platelet counts need only be maintained above $20 \times 10^9/l$ since severe haemorrhage is rare above this level (Serpick 1965; Editorial in *Brit. Med. J.* 1971).

Defects in the blood-clotting mechanism

The classical theory of blood clotting produced in 1904 stated that four components were involved: thromboplastin, calcium, pro-thrombin and fibrinogen. Little further progress was made in this ill-understood subject until 1947, when Owren in Norway dis-covered another component, factor V. Up to 1950, most of the work on blood clotting was carried out on what is now known as the extrinsic system and laboratory studies usually used the tissue factor, thromboplastin, to initiate clotting. It was thought that the reason why whole blood clotted after being withdrawn into a syringe was that thromboplastin was released from platelets or blood cells. About 1950, Macfarlane and his colleagues (see Macfarlane 1967 for a brilliant article on the subject) started to investigate clotting without the addition of any tissue factors. Their work provided a major contribution to the recognition and determination of the interaction of the five factors in the initial stages of the intrinsic system (factors XII, XI, IX, VIII and X on the new nomenclature). Unfortunately, the new factors initially brought new names and synonyms for each factor and there developed a complex scheme of factor interaction, so that only those working in the field could hope to understand the suggested clotting mechanism. Two innovations have, however, radically changed the situation, so that the basic mechanism and the principles of the blood-clotting tests can now be more readily followed. The first innovation is that the International Committee for Haemostasis and Thrombosis has assigned Roman numerals to the recognized blood-clotting factors, and the second is that Macfarlane (1964 and 1969) introduced a cascade theory for the interaction of the factors and suggested that each step in the sequence of events is an amplification stage. Each clotting factor is present in the plasma as a proenzyme and conversion of the proenzyme to the active enzyme occurs as a result of the splitting of a peptide bond, which brings about a conformational change in the molecule and reveals an active enzyme site. With the exception of factor XII, the splitting is brought about by the active enzymic form of the factor immediately preceeding it in the cascade. The clotting mechanism is divided into two systems.

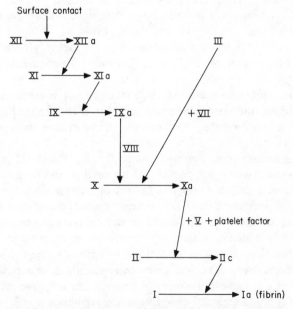

Fig. 6.5. Modification of Macfarlane's (1964, 1969) enzyme-cascade sequence of clotting reactions from surface contact to fibrin formation. The suffix 'a' denotes the active enzymatic form of each factor. The only major modification from the original is that factor IXa is now known to act directly on factor X, using factor VIII as a cofactor.

1   The *intrinsic system* has all the components present in the plasma. The sequence of action of factors in the intrinsic system is easy to remember as they are in descending order, except that factor X is misplaced. The sequence is XII, XI, IX (with VIII as cofactor), X, II and I, as illustrated in Fig. 6.5. Factor XII is activated by contact with collagen and basement membrane, as well as by foreign surfaces. The molecule is adsorbed to negatively charged surfaces, resulting in a conformational change and the appearance of an active enzymic site (factor XIIa). This enzyme then splits the proenzyme XI to form factor XIa, which then acts on IX to form IXa. In Macfarlane's original scheme, factor IXa then acted on VIII, but it is now known that IXa acts on X, using VIII as a cofactor. Factor Xa then acts on factor II (prothrombin) using factor V as a cofactor to form factor IIa (thrombin). Factor IIa splits several small negatively-charged peptide fragments from Factor I, thus removing repulsive forces from the molecule and allowing the remainder to polymerize and form the fibrin fibre. Finally, factor XIII, also present in the plasma, stabilizes and strengthens the fibrin polymers by forming covalent bonds between the fibrin chains (glutamic-lysine bridges).

The role of platelets in contact activation of factor XII and in the adsorption of factors VIII, IX, Xa and V has already been described.

The amplification factor at each stage is not known, but if it were tenfold, then each molecule of factor XII activated by contact with a foreign surface would result in one million molecules of fibrin.

2   The *extrinsic system* consist of two factors: factor III released by damaged tissues, and factor VII, present in the plasma as an inactive serine esterase enzyme. Following trauma, factors III and VII form a complex, factor VII becomes activated and then acts on X to form Xa. Both systems thus share a final common path (factor X, II and I). Calcium is required at several stages throughout the system but the exact sites of action need not be known. Recent observations have revealed extra interactions between various components, mainly in the form of positive and negative feedback systems; thus, factors activated late in the sequence potentiate the action of earlier stages (for instance, factor IIa potentiates the activation of factor Xa) and there are also inhibitors which prevent a local area of fibrin formation from becoming widespread. These details have as yet no clinical significance.

Six of the synonyms for the factors are still in general use and should be known. They are: anti-haemophilic globulin, VIII; Christmas factor, IX; prothrombin, II; thrombin, IIa; fibrinogen, I; fibrin 1a.

Tests for clotting defects

Once the basic sequence of events in clotting is understood the tests for defects become simple to understand. There are only two accurate basic tests which are widely used.

1 The *kaolin–cephalin time* which estimates the activity of the intrinsic system. This test is also known as the activated partial thromboplastin time; the only merit of this term is that it helps the laboratory specialist to confuse the non-specialist.

2 The *prothrombin time* which estimates the activity of the extrinsic system.

Clotting defects conveniently fall into two groups; in the first and by far the largest group are those patients with acquired deficiencies of several factors (II, VII, IX and X) resulting from treatment with coumarin drugs, vitamin K deficiency and liver disease. It can be seen from Fig. 6.5 that three of these factors lie in the extrinsic system and the specific test for the extrinsic system is the prothrombin time. In the second and much smaller group are those patients with congenital defects of one of the clotting factors. There are ten recognized congenital clotting defects, but 80–90% of the patients in this group are haemophiliacs (factors VIII deficiency), about 10–20% have factor IX deficiency, and only about 1% have deficiencies of one of the other eight factors. Thus, in practice almost all the congenital deficiencies are factors in the initial stages of the intrinsic system, and these can be detected by abnormalities in the kaolin–cephalin clotting test. By carrying out both the kaolin–cephalin time and the prothrombin time, it is therefore possible to determine whether the defect lies in the initial stages of the intrinsic system or in the components comprising the extrinsic system. If both tests are abnormal, then the defect is in the final common path or there are multiple abnormalities.

Test for intrinsic system

The simplest but least valuable test for the integrity of the intrinsic system is the whole blood-clotting time. Venous blood is taken and quickly placed in a glass tube at 37°C and observed at intervals until clotting occurs. Unfortunately, there is a wide range in the time taken for normal blood to clot by this method; it normally lies between 5 and 11 minutes, and in practice the whole blood-clotting time is found to detect only the grosser clotting defects with any degree of certainty. It is abnormally prolonged in many haemophiliacs but will only detect major deficiencies of factors VIII and IX. It is the method of choice in the control of heparin therapy (heparin is an inhibitor of factor IIa) as it is simple to carry out at the bedside and is sufficiently accurate for this purpose.

Kaolin–cephalin clotting time. The wide range of the whole blood-clotting time is due to two variables. First, activation of factor XII by the glass surface is variable and depends on such factors as the type of glass and how it has been washed. Secondly, there is a variation in the activity of the phospholipid factor supplied by the platelets, as platelet numbers vary considerably between individuals. The variation due to these two factors can be substantially abolished by the addition of kaolin and cephalin. Kaolin provides a maximal stimulus for factor XII activation and cephalin, an ether extract of human brain, is a platelet substitute. The suggestion that both kaolin and cephalin should be used in this way was made by Proctor & Rapaport in 1961 and the test is now widely used. The test is simple to carry out. Citrated plasma is obtained and to this is added a mixture of kaolin and cephalin followed by calcium, and the time taken for the mixture to clot is measured. Prolongation of the clotting time is almost always due to deficiency of factors VIII or IX (provided that deficiency of factor X onwards has been excluded by the prothrombin time) and the test is sufficiently sensitive to detect deficiencies of both these factors when their concentration is reduced to 30% or less of the normal value; that is, it will detect the mild haemophiliacs who only have severe bleeding after major surgical procedures.

If the kaolin–cephalin time is prolonged, it is possible to confirm the diagnosis of either factor VIII or IX deficiency if plasma is available from known cases of haemophilia and factor IX deficiency. Thus, if the addition of plasma known to be deficient only in factor VIII does not shorten the clotting time of the unknown sample from the patient under investigation, then the unknown must also have a deficiency of factor VIII. Specialized tests are also available for measuring fairly precisely the levels of factor

VIII and IX, expressed as a percentage of the normal value; these tests should always be carried out if they are available.

Test for the extrinsic system
The prothrombin time. The test used to measure the integrity of the extrinsic system is the one-stage prothrombin time. This test is carried out by adding factor III, which is present in tissue extracts, together with calcium to citrated plasma. Reference to Fig. 6.5 shows that factor III feeds into the intrinsic system at the stage X→Xa and hence prolongation of the prothrombin time results from deficiencies of I, II, V, VII and X. The prothrombin time is thus a misnomer since deficiency of at least five factors affects the test and prothrombin deficiency alone must be gross before the prothrombin time is prolonged. The test is chiefly sensitive to deficiency of factors V, VII and X. A deficiency of platelets does not affect the prothrombin time as the tissue extract containing factor III also contains the relevant phospholipid platelet clotting factor.

In all these clotting tests, it is necessary to determine the normal clotting time by using a normal plasma on each occasion that the test is carried out since there are always small differences in the activities of the reagents that are used.

Hereditary and congenital bleeding disorders
Blood clotting abnormalities can be conveniently divided into two categories, the congenital defects and the acquired defects. This section deals with those that are present from birth.

There is a group of patients who complain of excessive bleeding, either spontaneous or following trauma, usually starting early in life, and who frequently have a family history of a similar condition. These patients usually have one of three diseases, namely, haemophilia, factor IX deficiency or von Willebrand's disease. Out of 187 families with coagulation defects studied by Biggs & Macfarlane (1958), 138 had haemophilia, 20 had factor IX deficiency and 11 had von Willebrand's disease; the patients in the remaining 18 families either had rare deficiencies or had anticoagulants, or were not diagnosed.

Haemophilia (factor VIII deficiency)
The term haemophilia was first used by Schönlein in 1839 and applies to a life-long tendency to prolonged haemorrhage found

only in males and dependent on the transmission of a sex-linked abnormal gene. Apart from the demonstration by Addis in 1911 and Patek & Taylor in 1937 that an active fraction obtained from normal plasma and termed antihaemophilic globulin would shorten the clotting time of haemophiliac plasma, there was little understanding of the nature of the defect until the decade of 1950–60.

During this period it was found that there are in fact two diseases within the group of patients who on clinical and genetic grounds had been diagnosed as haemophilia: namely, patients with factor VIII deficiency and those with factor IX deficiency. As occurs only too frequently in medicine, this has led to confusion over terminology, and factor IX deficiency has been termed amongst others as haemophilia B and Christmas disease (after the name of the first patient). The simplest way out of this problem is to retain the term haemophilia for factor VIII deficiency, as this is the commonest deficiency, and to use the descriptive term 'factor IX deficiency' for the other disease. The growth of knowledge concerning factor VIII has led to the production of potent preparations and this has had a profound effect on the treatment and prognosis for the patient.

Deficiency of factor VIII results from a genetic defect on the X chromosome. The disease is thus almost entirely confined to males (XY) since the normal X chromosome in females is almost always capable of bringing about adequate factor VIII production. Females with haemophilia have been observed extremely rarely and these patients are either homozygous for the abnormal X chromosome or are heterozygous, but the normal X chromosome has not been adequate on its own to produce sufficient factor VIII. Daughters of males with haemophilia are obligatory carriers of the gene, since they must inherit the abnormal X chromosome. Sons, on the other hand, are always normal, since they inherit the Y chromosome. A female with a genetic defect on one X chromosome will transmit the disease to half her sons, and half her daughters will become carriers. Patients suspected of having haemophilia should be carefully questioned for a history of bleeding disorders occurring in the relations on the maternal side as opposed to the paternal side. It is possible that there is a steady spontaneous mutation rate of the gene responsible for factor XIII deficiency, since approximately one-third of all patients have no family history of the disease. The absence of family history may be due, however, to a lack of knowledge about the health of distant relatives.

The precise nature of the molecular defect in haemophilia has yet to be determined and there may be several different molecular defects giving the same disease characteristics, as is so often the case with hereditary disorders. Factor VIII is a large molecular complex containing two different types of molecules bound loosely together. The smaller molecule (coagulant factor, 120,000 MW) has the coagulant activity required as a cofactor in activation of factor X. This is the factor missing in haemophilia and its gene is present on the X chromosome. The other compound is a variable-sized polymer (up to 20×10^6 MW), the von Willebrand factor, whose function is to mediate platelet adhesion to subendothelial tissues. Its gene is on an autosomal chromosome. The coagulant activity can be measured biologically by its ability to act as a co-factor to factor IXa (Fig. 6.5); the von Willebrand factor can be measured by precipitation with specific antibodies.

In haemophilia, it has been found that although factor VIII coagulant activity is greatly depressed, the amount of von Willebrand factor is within normal limits. This observation is important, since it has been possible to make use of this difference for the detection of female carriers of haemophilia. Female carriers on average have half the clotting activity per unit of protein when compared to normals. Discrimination, however, is not perfect and about 10% of carriers fall within the normal range; thus, those with abnormal ratios can be definitely said to be carriers, but putative carriers with normal ratios cannot be definitely assured that they do not have the gene.

Clinical features. The characteristic clinical feature of severe haemophilia is the occurrence of spontaneous bleeding into joints and less frequently into muscles, these two sites accounting for about 95% of all bleeds requiring treatment (see Table 6.1). The presenting symptom is pain in the affected area and this can be very severe. Haemophiliacs rapidly become expert at diagnosing the onset of haemorrhage in its earliest stages, allowing treatment to be initiated at a time when it can be most effective. Bleeding into joints may occur weekly and, if not properly treated, results in crippling deformity. The knees, elbows and ankles are most commonly affected. Haematuria, epistaxis and gastrointestinal bleeding are less common. Intracranial bleeding is the commonest single cause of death, accounting for 25–30% of all deaths; only about one-half of the patients have a history of trauma (Eyster *et al.* 1978).

Table 6.1 Frequency of bleeding sites in 207 haemophiliacs. Adapted from Rizza (1977)

Lesion or operation	Percentage
Haemarthroses	79
Muscle haemotomas	15
Haematuria	
Epistaxis	
Gastrointestinal bleeding	each about 1–2%
Dental extraction	total 6%
Major surgery	

In a paper on the clinical management of haemophilia, Rizza (1977) relates the severity of bleeding and mode of presentation to the level of plasma factor VIII; this relationship is shown in Table 6.2. The severity of the disease often remains constant throughout a family.

The diagnosis of haemophilia is strongly suggested by the laboratory finding of a normal extrinsic clotting system (normal prothrombin time) and an abnormal kaolin–cephalin clotting time, since factor VIII deficiency is the commonest deficiency that is found in the initial steps of the intrinsic system. Confirmation can be obtained by showing that the addition of plasma from a known case of factor VIII deficiency to the patient's plasma does not correct the clotting defect or can be obtained by a specific assay of factor VIII concentration.

Treatment. Treatment may be therapeutic where there is either spontaneous bleeding from trauma, or it may be prophylactic if

Table 6.2 Relation between plasma factor VIII levels and severity of bleeding. Adapted from Rizza (1977)

Factor VIII level (units/100 ml)	Bleeding symptoms
50	None
25–50	Excessive bleeding after major surgery or serious accident (often not diagnosed until incident occurs).
5–25	Excessive bleeding after minor surgery and injuries.
1–5	Severe bleeding after minor surgery. Sometimes spontaneous haemorrhage.
0	Spontaneous bleeding into muscles and joints.

any type of operation is contemplated. The treatment consists of giving factor VIII in a concentrated form to maintain plasma factor VIII levels between 5 and 100% of normal, depending on the severity of the injury or extent of the surgical procedure. In general, the more extensive the bleeding or the degree of trauma, the larger the dose of factor VIII that is required. Two types of concentrated factor VIII preparations are available at the present time, cryoprecipitate and freeze-dried factor VIII. Cryoprecipitate, a relatively impure preparation which is nevertheless made in a simple manner by the freezing and slow thawing of plasma, is now being replaced by the more expensive but more highly purified freeze-dried material. The large amounts of factor VIII now being used by haemophilia patients has created problems of supply. It has been estimated that approximately 500,000 units of blood are required annually in the U.K., which is about 30% of the total number of units available.

One of the major advantages of the freeze-dried material is that adequate amounts can be injected in a small volume. This has made it possible for the patient to be treated at home, either by self-administration or by a competent person, thus allowing treatment to be carried out as soon as symptoms appear. This results in both rapid cessation of bleeding and rapid recovery. An excellent account of the value and advantages of home care can be found in the paper of Rizza & Spooner (1977).

After injection, factor VIII levels fall rapidly in the plasma and hence twice daily injections are necessary. The half-life in the plasma is about 8 hours. Frequent assays of factor VIII levels in the plasma may be necessary to ensure that the concentration is being maintained at the appropriate level.

Approximately 5–10% of haemophilic patients who are repeatedly injected with factor VIII develop antibodies which inhibit its functional activity. These patients require very large amounts of factor VIII, or recourse may have to be made to the use of factor VIII of bovine or porcine origin, but these can only be used for a short time, since antibodies to these molecules also develop rapidly.

Factor IX deficiency

The demonstration that there are two genetic defects giving rise to the clinical syndrome of 'haemophilia', was first clearly made by Biggs *et al.* in 1952, and was based on the observations that the addition of plasma from certain 'haemophiliacs' could correct the clotting defect in the plasma of other 'haemophiliacs', which could only be explained by postulating a deficiency of at least two factors. This second factor was soon identified as factor IX. The clinical features and inheritance are identical to factor VIII deficiency, but as a group the disease is milder. The incidence varies between different countries, but on an average about 20% of those with clinical 'haemophilia' have factor IX deficiency.

The diagnosis can be made by assay of factor IX level. Factor IX concentrate is available and it has been found that home treatment with factor IX given weekly or fortnightly as a prophylactic measure considerably reduces the incidence of haemorrhage (Rizza & Spooner 1977). Factor IX has a longer half-life in the plasma than factor VIII and hence can be given at less frequent intervals.

Von Willebrand's disease

This rare disease should be mentioned in a discussion on bleeding disorders since its frequency of occurrence in Britain is of about the same order as that of factor IX deficiency. It was first described by von Willebrand in 1926 as occurring in several families in islands in the Baltic (Åland Islands). It is characterized by excessive bleeding presenting in infancy which differs from haemophilia in that the defect is not sex-linked. The cause of bleeding is the failure of the platelets to form a haemostatic plug and this failure results from the reduction in the von Willebrand component of factor VIII. The von Willebrand factor is responsible for platelet adhesion to subendothelial tissues. As factor VIII is a complex molecule containing both the von Willebrand and coagulant proteins, a reduction in factor VIII coagulant is also found in this disease. Factor VIII concentration may be as low as 5–20% of normal (Abildegaard et al. 1968). This is similar in extent to that found in mild haemophilia. Thus, there is a reduction in both factor VIII coagulant activity and in the amount of the von Willebrand component, in contrast to the findings in haemophilia where only the coagulant activity is reduced.

An additional finding is that platelets fail to aggregate in the presence of the antibiotic ristocetin, in contrast to normal platelets. Although the physiological significance of this finding is not known for certain, it does correlate with the failure to form a haemostatic platelet plug. The test is, nevertheless, useful in diagnosis.

Most patients are probably heterozygous for the von Willebrand gene and the extent of the bleeding is not great, usually being confined to mucous membranes and skin, giving rise to epistaxes and ecchymoses. In some patients, more severe haemophilia-like bleeding is found, and these patients may be homozygous for the gene (Bloom & Peake 1977). Bleeding into joints does not occur but severe haemorrhage following surgical procedures is not uncommon. Apart from the factor VIII deficiency, the only abnormality that is consistently found is a prolonged bleeding time, although there may be periods when the test is within normal limits. The prolonged bleeding time distinguishes it from haemophilia and factor IX deficiency.

Deficiency of other clotting factors
Single deficiencies of factors other than VIII and IX are very rare, but all are found and all give rise to bleeding disorders with varying degrees of severity, except in the case of factor XII, which is not associated with excessive haemorrhage.

Acquired clotting defects
The blood clotting factors II, VII, IX and X are all produced in the liver and hence a deficiency in these factors occurs in liver disease. Moreover, the final stages in the synthesis of these factors involves a vitamin K-dependent carboxylase, which adds carboxyl (-COOH) groups to the proteins; these groups are necessary for the efficient functioning of the molecules. The coumarin drugs are vitamin K antagonists and their administration results in only partial carboxylation of the clotting proteins, with the result that they are considerably less active in the clotting cascade system. Similar results are found with vitamin K deficiency, which may be found in patients with intestinal malabsorption; it is also an additional cause of clotting-factor deficiencies in liver disease where there is biliary obstruction or fistula, since bile salts are required for vitamin-K absorption.

Examination of Fig. 6.5 shows that, except for factor IX, the clotting factors involved are in the extrinsic system and hence the test that is used for detecting these acquired deficiencies is the prothrombin time.

Investigation of a patient with abnormal bleeding
The diagnosis of bleeding due to thrombocytopenia is simple but the proper diagnosis and treatment of every patient with a coagu-

lant defect requires organization at the national level. This stems from the fact that some coagulation defects are extremely rare and that many of the tests are specialized and difficult to carry out reliably and accurately unless performed frequently. The most efficient way of overcoming this problem is to set up special laboratories for diagnosis. There are 42 Haemophilia Centres set up in Britain for this purpose and 4 centres, at Manchester, Oxford, Sheffield and London, are also major treatment centres. Nevertheless, since thrombocytopenia is one of the commonest causes of abnormal bleeding and since most of the congenital coagulation defects are due to either factor VIII or IX deficiency, the diagnosis can be made in most patients with reasonable certainty in any well-equipped laboratory.

Biggs (1968) has pointed out that there is no simple laboratory screening test that can be used to detect an abnormality. By far the most important requirement is a good history from the patient, who should be asked the following question (Biggs 1968).

'Has the patient ever bled excessively in the past and have any relatives bled excessively? More specifically, has the patient had tonsillectomy, major abdominal or orthopaedic surgery, or dental extractions in the past and if so, was there any abnormal bleeding?'

The excellent paper of Ingram (1977) should be consulted for a more detailed discussion on the taking of the patient's own, and family, history.

The few patients who give a history of excessive bleeding should then have the following tests performed.

> Bleeding time.
> Platelet count.
> Prothrombin time.
> Kaolin–cephalin clotting time.

If either clotting test is found to be abnormal, then making the exact diagnosis of the particular deficiency that is present will depend on the availability of plasma from patients with known deficiencies of factors VIII and IX (p. 112) and on the ability to perform accurately other tests that may be required.

It has been common to carry out bleeding times and whole blood-clotting times prior to operation in an attempt to detect those who may bleed abnormally. As Diamond & Porter (1958) have pointed out, these tests are totally inadequate in detecting abnormalities in every patient. All haemophiliacs have normal bleeding times and 20–30% of them have whole blood-clotting times within normal limits. There is no substitute for the procedure described above.

The fibrinolytic mechanism

The complex mechanism for producing fibrin is counterbalanced by a mechanism for the enzymatic lysis of clots. In order to explain the physiological function of the fibrinolytic system, it has been suggested, although not proved, that fibrin is slowly but continuously deposited on the vascular endothelium in order to seal off any deficiencies that may occur, and that the purpose of the fibrinolytic system is to remove the fibrin once it has served its function.

The dissolution of the fibrin into fibrin-degradation products (FDP) is carred out by the proteolytic plasma enzyme plasmin. Plasmin is present in the plasma in an inactive form (plasminogen) and must be converted into the active form by an activator, which is present in all tissues and is especially concentrated around blood vessels. Plasmin is not specific for fibrin, but will also break down into other protein components of plasma, including fibrinogen and the clotting factors V and VIII, and thus a mechanism is present which confines the activities of plasmin to fibrin alone (Fig. 6.6). The nature of this mechanism is still unknown, but a popular hypothesis postulates that when fibrin has been formed as the result of injury, plasminogen is absorbed on to the fibrin and is then converted to plasmin by the activator released from the damaged tissue. The plasmin can then digest the fibrin to which it is absorbed. Under normal conditions, any plasmin released from the fibrin into the circulation is immediately inactivated by combining with the plasma inhibitor, antiplasmin. In this way, generalized breakdown of fibrinogen and other proteins does not occur.

As well as tissue activator, physiological activators of plasminogen are also present in many body secretions, especially in urine (urokinase) and in the pleural and peritoneal cavities. Purified urokinase injected intravenously is a useful therapeutic agent for the treatment of various types of thrombosis. Non-physiological activators, such as streptokinase derived from certain streptococci, are also being used for this purpose.

Besides the physiological inhibitor of the fibrinolytic system, antiplasmin, there are several non-physiological inhibitors, of

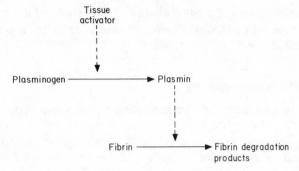

Fig. 6.6. The fibrinolytic mechanism. The continuous lines indicate conversion; the broken lines activity.

which ε-aminocaproic acid (EACA) and tranexamic acid are the best known. These inhibitors prevent the conversion of plasminogen to plasmin.

Disseminated intravascular coagulation

Disseminated intravascular coagulation describes a functional *process* (not a disease) in which there is a generalized activation of the clotting system followed by excessive activation of the fibrinolytic system as a secondary process.

Disseminated intravascular coagulation (DIC) is possibly most frequently seen associated with premature separation of the placenta, intrauterine death and with amniotic fluid embolism, and is also seen with certain bacterial infections (such as menigococcaemia, where the endotoxin causes widespread damage to vascular endothelium). It is a common complication following intravascular haemolysis of red cells after a mismatched transfusion. The syndrome also occurs occasionally after extensive accidental or surgical trauma, particularly following thoracic operation, and also follows the use of the artificial heart–lung pump. Other rare clinical associations are discussed by Deykin (1970).

In these diseases which are characterized by tissue injury and damage to vascular endothelium (in mismatched transfusion there is intravascular red-cell destruction), the clotting cascade sequence may be activated in one or both of two ways, namely, by the adsorption and activation of factor XII, and also by the release of factor III from the tissues or red cells. Dissemination of activated factor XII and factor III in the plasma leads to generalized fibrin deposition on vascular endothelium. If this is sufficiently exten-sive, there is a reduction of plasma fibrinogen concentration and also of other clotting factors, which impairs haemostatic activity. As the result of the fibrin formation, the fibrinolytic mechanism is activated by the absorption of plasminogen to the fibrin and its conversion to plasmin through the release of activator from vascu-lar endothelium and from the tissues. The plasmin then breaks down the fibrin into small fibrin-degradation products (FDP). When fibrin deposition is considerable, the activity of the plasmin results in high concentrations of FDP. This leads to further haemostatic impairment, since FDP inhibit fibrin clot-formation by interfering with the polymerization of fibrin monomer. The FDP also interfere with the aggregation of platelets, thus inhibiting their important physiological activity of plugging small vessels. The end result is generalized haemorrhage due to failure of the haemostatic mechanisms.

Clinical manifestation of the simultaneous activation of both clotting and fibrinolytic systems varies between patients and depends mainly on whether one system is activated more than the other by the tissue damage. Thus, if it is mainly the clotting mechanism which is activated, then the clinical picture is domi-nated by widespread thrombosis and infarction, but if the fib-rinolytic system dominates and the concentration of FDP rises to high levels, then the inhibition of fibrin polymerization and of platelet aggregation gives rise to generalized haemorrhage, which varies from petechiae and ecchymoses to bleeding from the uri-nary and gastrointestinal tract and may lead to death. Haemor-rhage may also occur into the pituitary gland, liver, adrenals and brain. Hypotension is commonly present and may be only mild but it can progress and become irreversible if not treated in time. Sometimes the activation of the two systems is so finely balanced that they cancel each other out and the patient is symptomless. This brief account is a simplification of the complex pathophysiol-ogy of the interaction between these two systems, of which the details are still in dispute. Further information may be obtained from the reviews of McKay (1968), Deykin (1970), and Sharp (1977).

Diagnosis

When the syndrome of disseminated intravascular coagulation is suspected to be present clinically, the diagnosis is frequently a matter of urgency and it is therefore the tests that can be carried out in the shortest time that are most frequently used. The most useful tests are:

1 *The platelet count.* Platelets become enmeshed in the fibrin clots on the vascular endothelium and thrombocytopenia is an early and very common sign.

2 The fibrinogen concentration, estimated as a *fibrinogen 'titre'* as follows. Serial dilutions of the suspected plasma are made and thrombin (factor IIa) added. Plasma with a normal fibrogen content will clot at a dilution of about 1 in 128, but only at higher concentrations (1 in 8 or 4 or may be non-clottable) when fibrinogen is depleted.

3 *The thrombin time.* When the fibrinogen concentration is normal, estimation of the thrombin time is a useful indication of the presence of excessive amounts of FDP. The thrombin time is carried out by adding thrombin to citrated plasma and measuring the time for the appearance of clotting. In the presence of FDP, the thrombin time is prolonged due to inhibition of fibrin polymerization.

4 *Estimation of FDP.* The presence of FDP can also be detected by a rapid immunological test using antibody specific against fibrinogen. If latex particles are coated with fibrinogen, they can be agglutinated by anti-fibrinogen and the addition of plasma containing FDP will inhibit this agglutination; the greater the FDP level, the greater the inhibition.

Treatment
Since the evidence indicates that the activation of the clotting system is the primary initiating stimulus and that fibrinolysis is mainly a secondary phenomenon activated for the most part as a consequence of fibrin formation, the treatment is aimed at preventing further coagulation by removal of the initiating cause (e.g. when it occurs in obstetric practice, rapid and non-traumatic vaginal delivery stops the clotting process). The most essential treatment in the acute bleeding state is transfusion with fresh blood or fresh-frozen plasma, not only to restore blood volume, but also to replace clotting factors. A fresh platelet transfusion may be necessary. Heparin (an antithrombin) can also be given, to prevent further fibrin formation, despite the presence of haemorrhage. The treatment that should only be used with caution is the administration of the plasminogen inhibitor ε-amino caproic acid

(EACA). There are recorded cases where the administration of EACA inhibited the fibrinolytic mechanism only to leave the clotting-cascade system to operate unopposed, with generalized and fatal thrombosis.

References

ABILDGAARD C. F., SIMONE J. V., HONIG G. R., FORMAN E. N., JOHNSON C. A. & SEELER R. A. (1968) Von Willebrand's disease. A comparative study of diagnostic tests. *J. Pediatrics*, **73**, 355.

ACKROYD J. F. (1962) The immunological basis of purpura due to drug hypersensitivity. *Proc. roy. Soc. Med.*, **55**, 437.

ADDIS T. (1911) The pathogenesis of hereditary haemophilia. *J. Path & Bact.*, **15**, 427.

ASTER R. H. (1972) Platelet sequestration studies in man. *Brit. J. Haemat.*, **22**, 259.

BIGGS R. (1968) The detection of defects in blood coagulation. *Brit. J. Haemat.*, **15**, 115.

BIGGS R., DOUGLAS A. S., MACFARLANE R. G., DACIE J. V., PITNEY W. R., MERSKEY C. & O'BRIEN J. R. (1952) Christmas disease: a condition previously mistaken for haemophilia. *Brit. Med. J.*, **2**, 1378.

BIGGS & MACFARLANE R. G. (1958) Haemophilia and related conditions: a survey of 187 cases. *Brit. J. Haemat.*, **4**, 1.

BLOOM A. L. & PEAKE I. R. (1977) Factor VIII and its inherited disorders. *Brit. Med. Bull.*, **33**, 219.

DEYKIN D. (1970) The clinical challenge of disseminated intravascular coagulation. *New Eng. J. Med.*, **283**, 636.

DIAMOND L. K. & PORTER F. S. (1958) The inadequacies of routine bleeding and clotting times. *New Eng. J. Med.*, **259**, 1025.

DOAN C. A., BOURONCLE B. A. & WISEMAN B. K. (1960) Idiopathic and secondary thrombocytopenic purpura: clinical study and evaluation of 381 cases over a period of 28 years. *Ann. Int. Med.*, **53**, 861.

EDITORIAL (1971) Platelet transfusions. *Brit. Med. J.*, **i**, 2.

EYSTER M. E. *et al.* (1978) Central nervous system bleeding in haemophiliacs. *Blood*, **51**, 1179.

GAYDOS L. A., FREIREICH E. J. & MANTEL N. (1962) The quantitative relation between platelet count and haemorrhage in patients with acute leukaemia. *New Eng. J. Med.*, **266**, 905.

HARKER L. A. & SLICHTER S. J. (1972) The bleeding time as a screening test for evaluation of platelet function. *New Eng. J. Med.*, **287**, 155.

HARRINGTON W. J., MINNICH V., HOLLINGSWORTH J. W. & MOORE C. V. (1951) Demonstration of a thrombocytopenic factor in the blood of patients with thrombocytopenic purpura. *J. lab. clin. Med.*, **38**, 1.

HESS A. F. (1914) Infantile scurvy: the blood, the blood vessels and the diet. *Medical Records N.Y.*, **86**, 990.

INGRAM G. I. C. (1977) Investigation of a long-standing bleeding tendency. *Brit. Med. Bull.*, **33**, 261.

LUSHER J. M. & ZEULZER W. W. (1966) Idiopathic thrombocytopenic purpura in childhood. *J. Pediatrics*, **68**, 971.

MACFARLANE R. G. (1964) An enzyme cascade in the blood-clotting mechanism, and its function as a biochemical amplifier. *Nature*, **202**, 498.

MACFARLANE R. G. (1967) Russell's viper venom. *Brit. J. Haemat.*, **13**, 437.

MACFARLANE R. G. (1969) The development of a theory of blood coagulation. *Proc. roy. Soc. B.*, **173**, 261.

McKAY D. G. (1968) Disseminated intravascular coagulation. *Proc. roy. Soc. Med.*, **61**, 1129.

MIELKE C. H., KANESHIRO M. M. & MAHER I. A. (1969) The standardized normal Ivy bleeding time and its prolongation by aspirin. *Blood*, **34**, 204.

MUSTARD J. F. & PACKHAM M. A. (1977) Normal and abnormal haemostasis. *Brit. Med. Bull.*, **33**, 187.

NAJEAN Y. & ARDAILLON N. (1971) The sequestration side of platelets in idiopathic thrombocytopenic purpura: its correlation with the results of splenectomy. *Brit. J. Haematol.*, **21**, 153.

PATEK A. J. & TAYLOR F. A. L. (1937) Hemophilia; some properties of substance obtained from normal human plasma effective in accelerating coagulation of hemophilic blood. *J. Clin. Invest.*, **16**, 113.

PROCTOR R. & RAPAPORT S. I. (1961) The partial thromboplastin time with kaolin. *Am J. clin. Path.*, **36**, 212.

RIZZA C. R. (1977) Clinical management of haemophilia. *Brit. Med. Bull.*, **33**, 225.

RIZZA C. R. & SPOONER R. J. D. (1977) Home treatment of haemophilia and Christmas disease: five years experience. *Brit. J. Haemat.*, **37**, 53.

SCHULMANN I. (1964) Management of idiopathic thrombocytopenic purpura. *Pediatrics*, **33**, 979.

SERPICK A. A. (1965) Platelet transfusion therapy. *J. Am. med. Ass.*, **192**, 625.

SHARP A. A. (1977) Diagnosis and management of disseminated intravascular coagulation. *Brit. Med. Bull.*, **33**, 265.

Recommended reading not mentioned in text

ESNOUF M. P. (1977) Biochemistry of blood coagulation. *Brit. Med. Bull.*, **33**, 213.

MACKIE M. J. & DOUGLAS A. S. (1976) Anticoagulants. *Brit. J. Hosp. Med.*, **16**, 118.

MARCUS A. J. (1969) Platelet functions I, II and III. *New Eng. J. Med.*, **280**, 1213, 1278 and 1330. (Review articles.)

PACKHAM M. A. & MUSTARD J. F. (1977) Clinical pharmacology of platelets. *Blood*, **50**, 555.

Objectives in learning: haemostasis

1 To know the morphology and function of platelets and the relationship between the number of platelets in the peripheral blood and the extent of abnormal bleeding.

2 To know about (a) the diseases associated with a failure of platelet production and (b) the disease associated with a shortened platelet life span, idiopathic thrombocytopenic purpura.

3   To know the cascade theory of the sequence of events in both the intrinsic and extrinsic clotting mechanisms.

4   To know the principles of the tests for the intrinsic system (whole blood-clotting time and kaolin–cephalin time) and for the extrinsic system (prothrombin time) in terms of the cascade theory.

5   To know the mode of inheritance, the mode of clinical presentation, the method of diagnosis and the treatment of haemophilia and factor IX deficiency.

6   To know the deficiencies in the acquired clotting defects due to coumarin drugs, vitamin-K deficiency and liver disease in terms of the cascade theory, and the method of diagnosis.

7   To know the principles of investigation of a patient suspected of having a haemostatic defect.

Chapter 7
Blood Transfusion

One of the main problems in the transfusion of blood is the avoidance of immunological reactions resulting from the differences in the chemical constituents of the red cells between donor and recipient. Blood groups have arisen because mutations have occurred in the genes controlling the surface constituents of the red cells. These alterations in the surface structures have not affected the function of the red cell but when the red cells of a donor are transfused into a recipient who lacks these surface structures, the recipient treats them as foreign substances and produces antibodies against them. There are at least a dozen major sites on the chromosomes where there are genes responsible for red-cell surface constituents and each of these sites is responsible for a different blood-group system. Although all the systems have given rise to transfusion difficulties (and in fact this is how many have been recognized), fortunately only two, the ABO and Rh systems, are of major importance and need be known by the student.

ABO system

The ABO system has three allelomorphic genes, A, B and O. The first two genes are responsible for converting a basic substance, H, present in every red cell, into A or B substances, thus converting the cells into groups A or B. The O gene has no known effect on the H substance, so that group O red cells simply contain H substance. H substance is a carbohydrate chain attached to lipid or protein in the red-cell membrane. A terminal polysaccharide unit is attached to this chain which determines the antigenic specificity, N-acetylgalactosamine in the case of A antigen and galactose in the case of B antigen. The A and B genes each code for the two different enzymes (glycosyltransferases) which attach these terminal groups. The O gene is an amorph and no glycosyltransferase is present. The three allelomorphic genes combine in pairs to give six possible genotypes, AA, AO, BB, BO, AB and OO. Be careful to distinguish between genotype and phenotype. Genotype refers to the specific genes that the person carries, whereas the phenotype refers to the observed characteristics. Determination of the blood group of a person is carried out using only two antibodies, anti-A and anti-B, but not with anti-O, since O substance does not exist. Since the presence or absence of H substance is not determined in routine blood grouping, genotypes can only be determined by family studies; e.g. the genotypes AO and AA cannot be distinguished by routine methods and both of these genotypes will be classified as the phenotype A. Thus, only four phenotypes are distinguished, namely A, B, AB and O. As the phenotype A includes the genotypes AA and AO, it follows that a mating between two people of phenotype A can produce a child of group O, if both parents are genotypically AO. The same principle holds for the phenotype B. (Note that it is a convention to print the genotype in italic and the phenotype in roman letters.)

The frequency of the ABO groups differs in different geographical regions but in Britain it is approximately: group O, 46%, A, 42%; B, 9% and AB, 3%.

There are several subgroups (such as A_1, A_2, etc.) within both the A and B groups, in which the basic A and B substances have minor biochemical changes. These are of considerable interest to the geneticist but are of no clinical significance. The antibodies anti-A_1 and anti-H are only very rarely found in patients requiring transfusion, and even when they are found, are usually too weak to lead to *in vivo* destruction of red cells containing A_1 or H substance.

Substances with antigenic properties closely similar to those of A and B are widely distributed in nature and are found in many animals and bacteria. Absorption of these substances from the gut is presumed to give rise to the production of anti-A and anti-B in the plasma of those who do not possess the substances on their red cells. Because of the presence of these antibodies it is necessary to transfuse blood with the same ABO group as that of the recipient. As group O cells do not react either with anti-A and anti-B, people of group O came to be known as universal donors. However, this is a dangerous concept, because group O people have anti-A and anti-B in their plasma, and in a small number of people these antibodies may be very potent so that a transfusion of 500 ml of group O blood may contain sufficient anti-A or anti-B to react with the recipient's cells and bring about their destruction. Group

O blood should be given to group A or B people only if the correct group is not available or if there is insufficient time to find out the group of the recipient.

Rh system

The Rh system derives its name from the findings of Landsteiner & Weiner (1940) that the antibody produced in rabbits by the injection of red cells from the Rhesus monkey would agglutinate 85% of human cells (Rh positive) but not the remaining 15% (Rh negative). It was quickly discovered that a similar antibody could also be found in the plasma of humans after blood transfusions and, most significant of all, it was also found in the plasma of mothers who had given birth to a child with haemolytic disease of the newborn. Several other antibodies were found in humans which were clearly recognizing antigens within the Rh system and in 1943 Fisher put forward the now well-known theory that there are three allelomorphic pairs of genes within the Rh system, C and c, D and d, E and e, each gene being responsible for producing a chemical substance on the surface of the red cell, C and c, D and d, E and e. The use of both capital and small letters to symbolize the genes and their respective end-products does not imply that one is dominant and one recessive.

People who were originally labelled as Rh positive on the old nomenclature have the D antigen on their red cells. Thus, people who are either homozygous DD, or heterozygous Dd, are Rh positive while those who are dd are Rh negative. The three genes on each chromosome (either C or c, D or d, E or e) are always inherited as a specific combination, the three commonest being CDe, cde, and cDE. As one of the chromosomes in each chromosome pair is derived from the father and one from the mother the final genotype might be CDe/cde which is the commonest combination. Rh-negative blood-transfusion donors are always cde/cde. The three genes are so close together on the chromosomes that no cross-over has ever been seen.

Differentiation of people into the Rh-positive and Rh-negative groups is carried out only with anti-D, since an anti-d has not yet been found. Use of an antibody of only one specificity means that homozygous DD people cannot be differentiated from heterozygous Dd people. However, since all the genes of the Rh system are inherited in specific combinations, determination of the pres-

ence or absence of the other antigens (C, c, E and e), especially
when combined with family studies, can almost always differentiate *DD* from *Dd*. This assessment is sometimes required to determine whether a Rh-negative mother who has anti-D in her plasma
can conceive a Rh-negative child by a Rh-positive father; this can
only happen if the father is *Dd*.

Clinically, only the D antigen and anti-D are important. The
reason for this is that the D antigen is a much more potent antigen
than the others (C, c, E or e) in the sense that it stimulates antibody production with far greater frequency than any of the other
antigens in the Rh system. Thus, a Rh-negative person (i.e.
cde/cde) has over a 50% chance of developing anti-D after the
transfusion of 1 unit of Rh-positive blood, whereas the 'c' antigen
will only provoke anti-c production in 2% of people lacking this
antigen (Mollison 1983). It is thus important that Rh-negative
people receive Rh-negative blood. On the other hand, the risk of
giving Rh-negative blood (*cde/cde*) to a Rh-positive person without the 'c' antigen (for instance, a recipient whose genotype is
CDe/CDe) is very small. Nevertheless, it should not be forgotten
that the 'c' antigen on Rh-negative red cells is capable of stimulating anti-c production in a few people and that this anti-c will not
only demand careful cross-matching at a subsequent transfusion,
but can cross the placenta and produce haemolytic disease of the
newborn in an infant with the 'c' antigen in its cells.

Other blood-group systems

Other blood-group antibodies which are sometimes a problem in
blood transfusions are the following: anti-K (Kell system), anti-Fy[a]
(Duffy system) and anti-Jk[a] (Kidd system). The names of the systems are derived from the people in whom the appropriate antibody was first detected. Unless there is an antibody against one of
the antigens in these systems present in the recipient, there is no
need to take these groups into account in selecting donor blood.
The chief reason for this is that the antigens of these sytems are
'poor' antigens and infrequently stimulate antibody production.
Thus, compared to the D antigen, their relative potency in
stimulating antibody production is 10–1000 times less. In most
hospital blood banks, it is now usual for the sera of all recipients to
be screened for the presence of one of these rarer antibodies. If
screening is not carried out, these antibodies will be discovered in

the final stages of a cross-matching procedure, using the antiglobulin test. When an antibody other than one belonging to the ABO system turns up in this way, first its specificity has to be identified and then the donor blood lacking the appropriate antigen must be found. As this takes a considerable time, cross-matching should always be carried out as far in advance as possible in order to allow for this complication.

Compatibility

The purpose of cross-matching blood before transfusion is to ensure there is no antibody present in the recipient's plasma which will react with any antigen on the donor's cells. The basic principle for doing this, i.e. agglutination of the red cells by antibody, has remained unchanged for over 100 years. The agglutination was first observed in 1875 by Landois, when he found that serum of one animal would agglutinate red cells of another species, although at that time it was not known that the agglutinating agents were antibodies, which were not discovered until 1890. However, there have been considerable advances in our techniques for making the agglutination technique more sensitive. The process of agglutination can be divided into two stages: (i) the reaction between antibody and the antigen on the red-cell surface; (ii) the clumping together of these red cells as a result of the antibody on their surface. Unfortunately, not all red-cell antibodies are able to bring about the second stage of agglutination without additional help and thus from a practical point of view, antibodies can be divided into agglutinating and non-agglutinating types. The ability of antibodies to agglutinate depends partly on the molecular structure of the antibody. Most IgM antibodies (i.e. those with a molecular weight of 900,000) can bring about agglutination, but only some IgG antibodies (molecular weight 160,000), notably anti-A and B, can bring about agglutination whereas most IgG antibodies do not do so. The Rh blood-group system would probably have been discovered long before 1940 if the IgG anti-D had been an agglutinating antibody. The non-agglutinating antibodies are sometimes referred to as 'incomplete'.

Three methods are available to convert non-agglutinating into agglutinating antibodies: namely, the addition of albumin, the use of enzymes, and the antiglobulin test. The addition of 20% albumin to the red-cell antibody solution or the treatment of red cells with proteolytic enzymes such as papain, will bring about agglutination in most instances. However, the most satisfactory test for the presence of non-agglutinating antibodies in a cross-match is the antiglobulin test.

The antiglobulin test

The antiglobulin test was first discovererd by Moreschi in 1908 but was forgotten and rediscovered by Coombs, Mourant & Race in 1945. At the time that the test was devised, antibodies were thought to be γ-globulins and the five classes of immunoglobulins IgG, IgM, IgA, IgD and IgE, had not then been identified. Under the new nomenclature, the basic constituent of an antiglobulin serum is anti-IgG. Anti-IgG is obtained by injecting human IgG into animals. Antiglobulin serum is able to bring about agglutination by combining with IgG antibodies on the red-cell surface. As anti-IgG antibodies are bivalent, they can combine with one IgG molecule on one red cell and with another IgG molecule on another cell and hence hold the red cells together as agglutinates.

The antiglobulin test can be used in two ways. It can be used to detect antibody already on the patient's cells *in vivo* as in types of acquired haemolytic anaemia and haemolytic disease of the newborn. Red cells from the patient or from cord blood are washed to remove free IgG, which would otherwise react with and neutralize the antiglobulin. After washing, antiglobulin serum is added and agglutination takes place (the direct antiglobulin test). Alternatively, the test can be used to detect the presence of non-agglutinating antibody in plasma or serum, as in the cross-matching of blood for transfusion. In this case, serum from the patient requiring tranfusion is incubated with red cells from the donor blood. Any antibody present in the recipient's serum which is active against the donor's cells will be absorbed on to the latter and after washing the cells, addition of antiglobulin serum will bring about agglutination (the indirect antiglobulin test).

Procedure for obtaining compatible blood

The ABO and Rh group of the recipient must first be determined. The ABO group is determined by the addition of agglutinating anti-A and anti-B to the red cells. Since it is so important to transfuse blood of the correct group, the grouping is checked by adding the patient's serum to known group A and B cells, since group A blood always contains anti-B in the plasma, group B blood has anti-A, and group O has anti-A and anti-B. The Rh group is determined using an anti-D serum with the indirect anti-globulin test.

Donor blood of the appropriate ABO and Rh group is then selected. The practice in England is for the organizations collecting the blood to determine the ABO and Rh group of the donor blood. Before this blood can be transfused, cross-matching must be carried out. The purpose of the cross-match is partly to ensure that there have been no errors in the original determination of the ABO group of the donor and recipient, and partly to ensure that no antibodies are present in the recipient which react with the donor's blood groups other than the ABO system. Since the antibodies in the recipient's plasma may be agglutinating or non-agglutinating two tests are carried out.

1   A test for agglutinating antibodies in which the patient's serum is added to the donor's cells and incubated at 37°C. The cells are then examined for agglutination.
2   A test for non-agglutinating antibodies, i.e. the antiglobulin test, using the patient's serum and the donor's cells.

Rh-negative donor blood is not always available for Rh-negative recipients and the question arises whether it is safe to give Rh-positive blood. Rh-negative males, especially elderly males, may receive Rh-positive blood provided care is taken to search for anti-D if subsequent transfusions are given. In women past the menopause the procedure is less safe because there is always the possibility, admittedly small, that she may have received a primary stimulus of D antigen from a Rh-positive fetus and the anti-D in the plasma may be below a detectable level. Transfusion of Rh-positive blood would then provoke a secondary response of anti-D production leading to a delayed transfusion reaction after a few days. Rh-positive blood must never be given to Rh-negative females of child-bearing age for fear of stimulating anti-D production and thus of producing haemolytic disease of the new-born in a subsequent pregnancy.

Ensuring that the patient receives the correct blood
Experience has shown that the most frequent cause of giving in-compatible blood is wrong labelling of samples, confusion between recipients with the same name, or failure to check from the label

on the bottle that it is the blood which has been cross-matched with the patient; it is only rarely due to mismatching of blood in the laboratory. Responsibility for giving the wrong blood usually lies either with the person who takes the sample of the recipient's blood for cross-matching or with the person who sets up the transfusion. When taking blood for cross-matching, great care should be taken that this is correctly labelled. The blood should be put into a container which is already labelled with the patient's name and *hospital number*. Requests for blood, however urgent, must be confirmed in writing. When the donor blood has been found to be compatible, the laboratory staff place a compatibility label on it, stating the patient's name, hospital number and the serial number of that particular bottle of blood. The person who sets up the transfusion is then finally responsible for ensuring that the patient's name and hospital number on the compatibility label apply to the patient who is being transfused and also that the serial number on the compatibility label is the same as the serial number of the bottle of blood. It cannot be too frequently emphasized that the commonest cause of incompatible transfusions is the carelessness of either registrar, houseman or nursing staff. A doctor or nurse must remain with the patient for 20 minutes following the start of the transfusion, to detect any evidence of a reaction due to incompatible or infected blood. This precaution is extremely important, since symptoms of an incompatible transfusion usually appear within this time and if the transfusion is stopped at this stage, the chance of a fatal outcome is reduced. These precautions and others together with the legal aspects of responsibility are discussed by James (1958).

Donor blood

Donor blood is obtained by the Regional Transfusion Centres administered by the Regional Hospital Boards. Donor blood (420 ml) is mixed with 120 ml of citrate–phosphate–dextrose, a solution found empirically to give good preservation of the blood. If the blood is stored at 4°C, 80% of the cells are still viable after 21 days, the remaining 20% being removed from the circulation by the reticuloendothelial system within a few hours of transfusion. After 21 days of storage the percentage of viable cells falls off rapidly, so that the blood is not used after this period of time. Another reason for not using blood beyond this storage period is that should bacterial contamination have occurred during the taking of the blood, the longer it is stored, the more likely it is that bacterial growth will have proceeded to such an extent that a severe transfusion reaction ensues.

Hazards of blood transfusion

Blood transfusion has become such a commonplace procedure (there is about one transfusion for each hospital bed each year in Britain) that the hazards of transfusion are frequently overlooked. The actual mortality resulting directly from transfusion is difficult to estimate and undoubtedly varies from region to region. The main cause of death nowadays is post-transfusion hepatitis; incompatible transfusion, bacterial infection, circulatory overload and other causes are only to blame in the minority of cases. In those regions where there is a high incidence of hepatitis-virus carriers, the mortality rate could be as high as one for every 1000 transfusions (Moore 1952).

The unfavourable reactions to transfusion are either immediate, in which case they are due to pyrogens, allergens, bacteria, circulatory overloading or incompatible blood, or the reactions are delayed, in which case they are due to the transmission of diseases, such as hepatitis, malaria and syphilis.

The recognition of these hazards has been a lengthy process. Before the discovery of the ABO blood groups, haemolytic reactions due to this blood-group system were frequent and hence transfusions were few in number. When ABO incompatibility had been eliminated one of the first hazards to be recognized was the transfer of syphilis and with the increasing use of blood after the introduction of citrate as an anticoagulant in 1914, reactions due to allergens and pyrogens became recognized. It was in 1943 that the first reports of transmission of hepatitis were made (Ministry of Health Memorandum 1943) and it was during this and the following decade that reactions due to blood groups other than the ABO group were described.

Haemolytic reactions due to incompatible blood

With the recent advances in blood-grouping techniques, haemolytic reactions have now become rare; Ramgren et al. (1958) assessed the incidence in Sweden to be about 1 in 5000 during the 5 years 1951–55. Mollison (1979), surveying more recent figures, came to a similar conclusion. The number of mismatched transfusions, however, is certainly greater than this, since the distribution of the ABO groups is such that, if either donor or recipient is mis-identified and the wrong blood given, there is only a 1 in 3 chance of that blood being incompatible (e.g. a group A recipient mis-identified as group O and receiving group O blood, would not have a haemolytic reaction, whereas the reverse would lead to incompatibility). This means that the incidence of mismatched (but not necessarily incompatible) transfusion may be as high as 1 in 1500.

The symptoms that are found after a transfusion of incompatible blood depend on whether there is intravascular lysis of the transfused cells or whether they are removed by the reticuloendothelial system without initial lysis. Intravascular lysis, haemoglobinaemia and haemoglobinuria are almost always due to the action of anti-A or anti-B which bring about lysis in conjunction with the complement system. Usually within a few minutes of transfusing ABO incompatible blood, there is a feeling of heat along the vein used for transfusion, flushing of the face, pain in the lumbar region and chest, and chilliness. This is followed by fever. These effects are thought to be due to the release of the complement fragments C3a and C5a, since the complement sequence is known to be activated following the combination of anti-A with A red cells. If the reaction is severe, there is circulatory collapse and sometimes extensive haemorrhage due to the release of clotting factor III and plasminogen activator from red cells, which results in disseminated intravascular coagulation and fibrinolysis (p. 122). If the patient survives the initial reaction, there is about a 10% chance of developing oliguria or anuria. The mechanism by which this is brought about is still disputed, but it is probable that an important factor is the toxic action of high concentrations of haemoglobin on the renal tubes. The immediate treatment of a mismatched transfusion whould therefore be to promote diuresis with mannitol followed by sodium bicarbonate (Barry & Crosby 1963). When deaths do occur, they are usually the result either of the disseminated intravascular coagulation or of the renal failure. If the latter is correctly treated with due attention to water, electrolyte and protein metabolism, the mortality should be negligible. The mortality following ABO incompatibility is probably of the order of 10%. Wallace (1977) reported 4 deaths from 40 incompatible transfusions in a survey involving 130,000 recipients of blood.

When blood transfusion is followed by extravascular destruction of red cells there are usually only chills and fever occurring 1 or more hours after the start of the transfusion. The most common antibody causing extravascular destruction is anti-D. This type of incompatibility is almost never followed by renal failure.

Another type of incompatibility is the delayed haemolytic transfusion reaction. This occurs when a recipient has been previously immunized by transfusion or pregnancy but in whom the antibody in the plasma has become too weak to be identified. Following the transfusion, a secondary immunological response takes place and the antibody titre rapidly rises, bringing about haemolysis, usually about 7 days later. Typically, the patient develops anaemia, fever, jaundice and sometimes haemoglobinuria. The incidence of this type of reaction may be as high as 1 in 4000 recipients (Pineda *et al.* 1978).

Pyrexia due to pyrogens
Pyrogens were once a common cause of reactions. They are soluble polysaccharides produced by bacteria and are present in preparations of distilled water, citrate, dextrose and sodium chloride. Contamination by pyrogens has been reduced by strict control during manufacture of the anticoagulants. Chills and fever start 30–60 minutes after the onset of the transfusion and can be mitigated or abolished by aspirin. Since pyrogen reactions are now a rarity, febrile reactions should always suggest the possibility that incompatible red cells or leucocytes have been transfused.

Allergic reactions
Allergic reactions were found to occur in 3% of transfusions by Stephen *et al.* (1955). These reactions are the fault of recipients who possess antibodies (immunoglobulin class IgE, or skin-reacting antibodies) to allergens present in the donor's plasma. Stephen *et al.* (1955) stated that the criteria for allergic reactions were the development of urticarial wheals, erythema, maculopapular rash, or oedema around the eyes. In some patients there is an accompanying fall in blood pressure, which can endanger life. Bronchial spasm and laryngeal oedema are rare. The symptoms of allergic reactions can be relieved by the administration of adrenalin in the severe cases and antihistamines in the mild cases.

Infected blood

Transfusion of infected blood is fortunately rare, but when it does occur is frequently lethal. The low incidence is due entirely to the most painstaking precautions to keep solutions, storage containers and transfusion equipment sterile. However, there is one source of infection that is difficult to eliminate and that is the introduction of organisms from the skin during blood donation, despite careful attempts to disinfect the skin. Skin contaminants entering donor blood are usually staphylococci which fortunately do not grow at 4°C; as many as 2% of all donor blood may be found to have these organisms within the first 24 hours, but they are killed off during storage and are only rarely found after 3 weeks' storage.

Occasionally, however, Gram-negative bacteria of the type found in faeces and dirt enter into donor blood and these will grow slowly at 4°C (doubling-time about 8 hours) although they grow preferentially at 20°C. In 2–3 weeks at 4°C, growth can be sufficient to cause a lethal reaction and it is usually this type of organism that is found in the fatal cases. The growth rate of these bacteria is considerably speeded up if the blood is brought to room temperature. The risks of transfusing infected blood can thus be minimized by keeping blood at 4°C until the moment of transfusion and by using blood stored for not more than 3 weeks. Once a blood container has been opened for cross-matching or for preparing concentrated red cells it must be used within 24 hours. One or more deaths from infected blood are usually reported each year in the U.K. The chief signs of transfusions of infected blood are the rapid onset of pyrexia and circulatory collapse.

Circulatory overload

Circulatory overload with consequent cardiac failure can easily be brought about by the too rapid transfusion of blood, especially in the elderly and in those who have been severely anaemic. The first signs are dyspnoea, a dry cough, moist rales at the lung bases, and a rise in jugular venous pressure. If there is any indication of overload, the transfusion must be stopped and venesection may be necessary. The risk of circulatory overload can be minimized in patients with severe anaemia by giving only 250 ml of concentrated red cells (i.e. a unit of blood with most of the plasma-citrate removed) and restricting the rate of transfusion to 1 ml/kg body weight/hour. If the patient is only mildly anaemic and has a normal cardiac function, 1000 ml can be safely transfused over a

5-hour period. This is about one drop/second with the standard giving sets.

Citrate toxicity

Citrate toxicity may develop and can cause death if the blood has to be given very rapidly. It is due to the reduction in ionized calcium in the patient's plasma. The signs are gross skeletal muscle tremors and prolongation of the QT interval in the ECG. If more than 2 litres are given every 20 minutes then each litre should be accompanied by 1 g of calcium gluconate. The potassium which leaks out of red cells during storage is probably only dangerous when excess citrate is present in the recipient's plasma.

Transmission of disease

Post-transfusion hepatitis

Virus hepatitis is the most important complication of the transfusion of blood because of the high incidence of virus carriers in the population, the length of the illness and the high fatality rate. It has been estimated that there may be 30,000 cases of clinical post-transfusion hepatitis in the U.S.A. each year and about 1500–3000 cases are thought to be fatal.

Several viruses are known to cause hepatitis, namely hepatitis A and hepatitis B, cytomegalic virus, herpes simplex virus, Epstein–Barr virus and an unidentified virus (or group of viruses) termed for convenience 'non-A, non-B'. Of this collection of viruses, it is only the HB and the non-A, non-B which play any significant part in post-transfusion hepatitis, since it is only these viruses which exist in the carrier state in asymptomatic blood donors.

Knowledge of the hepatitis B virus has been greatly expanded since the discovery that the abnormal serum protein known as Australia antigen (first found in the serum of an Australian aborigine) is the excess surface coat of the HB virus. The virus has been identified by electron microscopy as a 42 nm particle (the Dane particle) and its presence in serum can be identified by a sensitive radioimmmunoassay test, involving the use of an antibody against the surface antigen, anti-HBsAg. The prevalence of HB virus in symptomless carriers (as recognized by finding the presence of HBsAg) varies between different populations, being as low as 0·1% in volunteer donors in the U.K. and U.S.A. and as high as 10% in paid donors in the U.S.A. The usual mode of transmission of the virus in the general population is not known. It has been suggested that it is a sexually transmitted disease, as the virus has been found in vaginal secretions. The elimination of all donor blood containing detectable HbsAg has brought about a very considerable reduction in the incidence of hepatitis due to the HB virus. The sensitivity of the tests, however, is probably not sufficient to eliminate all carriers.

Very little is known about the non-A, non-B virus and, as its name implies, its presence is recognized by exclusion of known viruses and it has not yet been identified. Its prevalence appears to be low in the U.K. and its highest incidence, as with the hepatitis B virus, appears to be in paid donors. The existence of the virus has been recognized in many countries, and is an important cause of hepatitis in the U.S.A. This is exemplified by the findings of Seef *et al.* (1977) who found in a study of patients receiving transfusion in the years 1969–1973 that the total incidence of transfusion hepatitis was 10·9%, but that only a quarter of these were due to the HB virus. In a later study between 1973 and 1975, when all donors identified as carrying HB virus had been eliminated, the incidence of hepatitis was still about 10%, none of which could be ascribed to the hepatitis B virus and was therefore presumed to be non-A, non-B (Seef & Wright 1978). The incidence of hepatitis was high in this study because well over half the patients received blood from paid donors. Nevertheless, in the U.S.A. the non-A, non-B virus may well be the cause of hepatitis in 80–90% of those who receive transfusions of volunteer donor blood which does not contain HBsAg, as determined by radioimmunoassay.

A British prospective survey, carried out in London in 1969–1971, found a lower incidence of transfusion hepatitis than in the U.S.A. survey, namely, about 1%, which was similar to the 0·8% of icteric hepatitis found in a previous British survey carried out in the Liverpool area in 1949. Of the 768 transfused patients who were followed up for 6 months, 8 developed hepatitis, 5 were icteric and 2 died. The mortality rate was equivalent to about 1 death for each 1000 units transfused.

It can be seen from Fig. 7.1, that the time of onset of overt hepatitis varies from about 2 weeks to 6 months after the transfusion. For every case of icteric hepatitis, it is generally accepted that there are several times as many cases of anicteric hepatitis. Thus, most of those who develop the disease are only mildly ill or

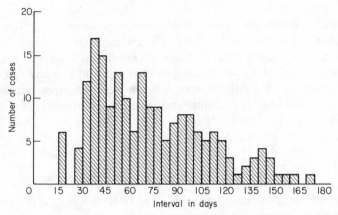

Fig. 7.1. The interval from transfusion to onset of hepatitis in 195 patients receiving blood or blood products on a single day. Adapted from Mosley (1965).

may have no symptoms. The hepatitis can only be recognized in these patients by a rise in the plasma levels of liver enzymes, such as alanine transminase. A small number of patients suffer considerable liver damage with a rise in serum bilirubin levels. The mortality rate almost certainly varies with the strain of the virus. Thus, in some outbreaks in renal dialysis units involving hepatitis B, the mortality following accidental infection in the attending staff has been over 50%. In the U.K. survey of 1974, it was 25%, although the numbers involved were small. Mosley (1965) reported an 11% mortality in those who developed icteric hepatitis, whereas Seef *et al*. (1977) reported only one death in 40 patients with raised serum bilirubin levels. In this latter group, the virus was mainly non-A, non-B, which may therefore be less virulent. Nevertheless, although non-A, non-B may have only a low immediate mortality, Seef & Hoofnagle (1977) found that approximately 10% of those infected with this virus develop a chronic active hepatitis, confirmed by liver biopsy.

A WHO report (1970) estimated that removal of all blood donors with HbsAg would only reduce the incidence of hepatitis by 25%. Thus, it follows that until we have reliable methods for determining all types of virus, the only way to minimize the morbidity and mortality is the avoidance of unnecessary transfusions.

Other diseases

Other diseases that have been known to be transmitted by transfusion are syphilis and malaria. The prevention of transmission of syphilis is by serological testing of all donors although this will not demonstrate all those infected, since it is possible to have syphilis with negative serological tests. Another factor of importance is the storage of blood at 4°C since spirochaetes do not survive for more than a few days under these conditions. Donors with a history of malaria are not accepted.

Procedure in the case of transfusion reactions

In the majority of instances it is easy to diagnose the type of transfusion reaction. Allergic reactions are obvious and only require antihistamines. Symptoms occurring within 20 minutes of starting a transfusion are always due to incompatibility or infected blood and clearly the transfusion must be stopped. It is the occurrence of rigors and fever after 30–60 minutes which causes difficulty in the diagnosis, since some of these reactions are due to bacterial pyrogens, and some are due to incompatibility. In these patients with delayed symptoms, the transfusion should be temporarily stopped, the blood being replaced with saline, and the patient warmed. If symptoms do not rapidly disappear, the transfusion should be abandoned and the reaction investigated further. Fortunately mild reactions of this type due to incompatibility are only rarely fatal.

Investigation of a transfusion reaction due to incompatibility

There are two problems to elucidate after a suspected transfusion of incompatible blood. First, the demonstration that destruction of red cells has in fact taken place, and secondly, which antigen–antibody system was involved.

Immediately the transfusion has been stopped, a blood sample is obtained and centrifuged; the plasma is examined for the presence of free haemoglobin and the plasma bilirubin concentration is estimated. A urine sample is also examined for the presence of haemoglobin. If incompatible cells are still present in the recipient's circulation, their presence can often be detected by serological methods. Thus, the presence of group A cells in a group O patient can be detected by the addition of anti-A which will agglutinate only A cells in the sample.

The ABO and Rh group of both the recipient and donor are checked and a cross-match repeated using the serum obtained from the recipient prior to transfusion. These tests will reveal whether the incompatibility is within the ABO system or whether it involves the D antigen of the Rh system. If the ABO and Rh (D) groups were compatible, but the cross-match shows the presence of an antibody, the specificity of the antibody can be identified by further testing against a panel of red cells of known blood-group specificity.

The remains of the donor blood in the pack after every transfusion should be kept at 4°C for 24 hours so that any adverse reaction can be adequately investigated.

References

BARRY K. G. & CROSBY W. H. (1963) The prevention and treatment of renal failure following transfusion reactions. *Transfusion*, **3**, 34.

JAMES J. D. (1958) *Practical Blood Transfusion*. Blackwell Scientific Publications, Oxford.

LANDSTEINER K. & WIENER A. S. (1940) An agglutinable factor in human blood recognizable by immune sera for Rhesus blood. *Proc. soc. exp. Biol. (N.Y.)*, **43**, 223.

Ministry of Health Memorandum (1943) Homologous serum jaundice. *Lancet*, **i**, 83.

MOLLISON P. L. (1983) *Blood Transfusion in Clinical Medicine* (7th edn). Blackwell Scientific Publications, Oxford.

MOLLISON P. L. (1979) Some clinical consequences of red cell incompatibility. *J. Roy. Coll. Physicians*, **13**, 15.

MOORE C. V. (1952) Medical problems created by a National Blood Transfusion Program. *J. Am. med. Ass.*, **149**, 1613.

MOSLEY J. W. (1965) The surveillance of transfusion-associated viral hepatitis. *J. am. med. Ass.*, **193**, 1007.

PINEDA A. A., TASWELL H. F. & BRZICA S. M. (1978) Delayed haemolytic transfusion reactions. An immunologic hazard of blood transfusion. *Transfusion Philad.*, **18**, 1.

RAMGREN O., SKOLD E. & TANBERG J. (1958) Immediate non-haemolytic reactions to blood transfusion. *Acta med. Scand.*, **162**, 211.

SEEF L. B. & 13 others. (1977) A randomized, double blind controlled trial on the prevention of post-transfusion hepatitis. *Gastroenterology*, **72**, 111.

SEEF L. B. & HOOFNAGLE J. (1977) Leader. *Annals of Internal Medicine*, **86**, 818.

SEEF L. B. & WRIGHT E. C. (1978) in Internationl Forum Discussion. *Vox Sang.*, **32**, 346.

STEPHEN C. V., MARTIN R. C. & BOURGEOIS-GAVARDIN M. (1955) Antihistaminic drugs in treatment of non-haemolytic transfusion reactions. *J. Am. med. Ass.*, **158**, 525.

WALLACE J. (1977) *Blood Transfusion for Clinicians*. Churchill Livingstone, Edinburgh.

WORLD HEALTH MEMORANDUM (1970) *Bulletin of the World Health Organization*, **42**, 957.

Recommended reading not mentioned in text.

ROBERTS R. (1960) *An Introduction to Human Blood Groups.* Heinemann, London.

Objectives in learning: blood transfusion

1   To know about the inheritance of the ABO system, and the type and distribution of associated antibody.

2   To know the distribution and mode of inheritance of the D antigen of the Rh system.

3   To know the principles involved in the selection of donor blood of suitable ABO and Rh groups for a recipient, and the principles of the cross-match, including the antiglobulin test.

4   To know the hazards of blood transfusion (incompatible blood, pyrogenic and allergic reactions, bacterial infection, citrate toxicity, and transmission of disease).

5   To know how to investigate a patient suspected of receiving an incompatible transfusion.

Chapter 8
Haemolytic Disease of the Newborn

Haemolytic disease of the newborn is the result of the transplacental passage of maternal blood-group antibodies, which become attached to the fetal cells and cause their destruction. In almost all cases, the antibody concerned is within the Rh blood-group system. Giblett (1964) found that 93% of the cases were due to anti-D, 6% to anti-c, or anti-E, and only the remaining 1% were due to antibodies of other blood-group systems, including the ABO system. Without treatment, the mortality rate of affected infants is about 20%, but the antenatal prediction of the disease, together with the introduction of treatment by exchange transfusion has considerably reduced the mortality rate. Approximately 60% of affected infants require an exchange transfusion and in the best hands efficient treatment results in the survival of about 95% of all those who are born alive. Nevertheless, during the decade 1958–68, the disease resulted in about 300–400 neonatal deaths each year in Britain and approximately an equal number were stillborn. The introduction during 1968 of prophylactic injections of anti-D into the mother immediately after labour to prevent active immunization (p. 152) means that haemolytic disease due to anti-D will become a rarity in about 20 years' time. Nevertheless, it is most important that antenatal prediction of the occurrence of the disease should continue to be made, since it is unlikely that complete suppression of immunization can be brought about. A low mortality rate can only be maintained if those who are born with the disease are treated within a few hours of birth. Once an Rh-negative mother (genotype *cde/cde*) has anti-D in her plasma there is no known way of inhibiting this production and all subsequent Rh-positive infants (those with the *D* gene) will be affected.

Haemolytic disease due to anti-D
The discovery of the aetiology of this disease is described in the classical paper of Levine *et al.* (1941).

The Rh antigens are only present on red cells and it is the

passage of red cells from the fetus across the placenta into the mother that gives rise to the immunization of the mother in the first place. Direct evidence for the presence of fetal red cells in the maternal circulation has been obtained using the acid-elution (Kleihauer) technique in which a dried film of maternal blood on a glass slide is dipped into a buffer solution at pH 3·5. Adult haemoglobin is soluble in this solution but fetal haemoglobin is not, so that subsequent counter-staining demonstrates the intact fetal red cells amongst a background of pale haemoglobin-free maternal cells (Plate 7). Fetal cells can occasionally be found in the maternal circulation during pregnancy, especially during the third trimester, but transplacental passage occurs mainly at the time of labour. About 15% of women have been shown to have more than 0·1 ml of fetal red cells in the circulation after labour and occasionally the number of cells may exceed 50 ml. There is evidence that the greater the number of fetal cells in the circulation after labour, the greater the chance of developing antibodies (Clarke 1967, 1968). Relationship between the total amount of fetal red cells in the maternal circulation immediately after labour and the incidence of immunization of mothers 6 months later is shown in Table 8.1.

In a Caucasian population, about 17% of the women are Rh-negative. The fathers of the children born to these mothers will be either homozygous DD, heterozygous Dd, or dd, and it can be calculated that only about 50% of all mothers who are Rh-negative will give birth to 2 successive Rh-positive infants. In theory then, the incidence of HDN should be 8% of all second pregnancies, but in practice the incidence was only about 1% before the advent of preventive therapy (see p. 152). This results from the fact that frequently the amount of fetal red cells crossing the placenta is insufficient to initiate immunization, combined with the fact that

Table 8.1 Relationship between total fetal red cells in the maternal circulation after labour and subsequent immunization of mother. Adapted from Clarke (1968)

Estimated number of fetal red cells (ml)	0	0·02	0·04	0·06–0·08	0·1–0·2	0·22–0·78	>0.8
Incidence of immuniz-ation (%)	3·7	4·5	10·3	14·6	18·7	21·1	23·5

only some 60–70% of mothers are able to respond to the D-antigen by producing anti-D.

It is very unusual for the first-born child to be affected with HDN, the incidence being slightly less than 1% of all Rh-negative mothers with no history of transfusion or abortion. The reason for this is that it is only occasionally that significant numbers of fetal red cells cross the placenta sufficiently early in pregnancy to stimulate anti-D production before the child is born. The total incidence of HDN in first born children is nevertheless higher than 1%, as a number of mothers become immunized through abortion or miscarriage or by transfusion of Rh-positive blood.

If the fetal red cells in the mother after labour bring about a primary immunization, antibody may be detected within the following 6 months. In about half the cases, however, antibody concentrations do not rise sufficiently high for anti-D to be detected at this time by the antiglobulin test. During the subsequent pregnancy with an Rh-positive fetus, a few fetal red cells crossing the placenta early in pregnancy provide a secondary stimulus to anti-D production, which can usually be detected by the 28th week but may not appear until the last few weeks of pregnancy.

Anti-D is found amongst both the IgM and IgG classes of immunoglobulin. Only some mothers have IgM anti-D, but all mothers have IgG anti-D. It is the IgG class that is actively transferred across the placenta to the fetus.

Mothers who lack the c or E antigens, for example, those whose genotype is *CDe/CDe*, can produce anti-c or anti-E if red cells containing the C or E antigens cross the placenta. The incidence of these antibodies is low and if they are to be detected antenatally, it is necessary to look for them in both Rh-positive and negative mothers. Since this involves a great deal of laboratory work, it is only carried out at a few centres.

Clinical features

There is a very great variation in the severity of the disease in the child. At one end of the scale there are infants who are not anaemic at all at birth and who never become jaundiced. However, the haemoglobin concentration of these infants may fall more rapidly than is normally found after birth and values as low as 6 g/dl may be found up to 30 days later. All infants with antibodies on their red cells (positive antiglobulin test) should therefore be followed up for 1 month after birth.

The first affected child in a family is usually less severely affected than later children, probably because the anti-D concentration in the mother is lower with the first child than subsequently. The overall severity of the disease in a family when several infants are affected tends to be consistent, the infants are either all mildly or all severely affected, although there are exceptions.

Moderately severely affected babies may or may not be anaemic at birth, but the rate of red-cell destruction is such that jaundice develops within a few hours. Jaundice is not seen at the time of birth since prior to this the bilirubin is excreted by placental transfer. Within 48–72 hours of birth, the plasma bilirubin may rise to 350–700 μmole/l. The rate of rise of plasma bilirubin is governed partly by the rate of red-cell destruction and partly by the degree of maturity of the bilirubin excretory mechanism, that is, on the state of development of glucuronyl transferase. As a result of the poor development of the excretory mechanism for bilirubin in many infants, it is quite common for the child with a cord haemoglobin within the normal range (lower limit 13·5 g/dl) to become severely jaundiced. The danger associated with a high bilirubin level is the development of kernicterus with its attendant brain damage, characterized by spasticity, arched back and death from respiratory failure. Those that survive usually have a subnormal intelligence.

The most severely affected infants become so anaemic that they develop cardiac failure and are either stillborn or die shortly after birth, although those with mild cardiac failure can be resuscitated by exchange transfusion. Apart from anaemia, the characteristic feature of these children is oedema. The stillbirth rate is approximately 15% of all infants with haemolytic disease and death may occur from the 20th week onwards.

Haemolytic disease due to anti-A and anti-B

Haemolytic disease due to the ABO blood group is almost entirely confined to group A and B infants born to Group O mothers, since some group O mothers have anti-A and anti-B of the IgG class of antibodies which is the type which crosses the placenta. Mothers of group A and B usually have only IgM anti-B and anti-A respectively and this large molecule does not cross the placenta. The disease is possibly as common as that due to anti-D, but it is rarely recognized since it is usually very mild; severe anaemia is uncommon and the child rarely requires treatment by exchange transfusion. Part of the difficulty in recognizing the disease is that the antiglobulin reaction carried out on the cord cells is usually negative or only very weak. Two fairly consistent findings are an increase in osmotic fragility of the red cells and the presence of spherocytes in cord blood.

Management of mother and child

It is vitally important to predict antenatally the birth of an affected infant so that labour can take place in a hospital equipped to carry out exchange transfusion within the first few hours of life. Rh-negative mothers must therefore be examined for the presence of anti-D in their plasma during pregnancy. The ABO and Rh blood groups of all pregnant mothers are determined early in pregnancy, and all those who are Rh-negative are examined for the presence of anti-D at 12 weeks. Any anti-D present at this time was probably initially produced during or soon after the previous pregnancy. A further examination is carried out at 28 weeks. This time is chosen because if anti-D is present, this is also the optimum time for carrying out amniocentesis for the antenatal determination of the severity of the disease.

A method of predicting the severity of the disease would be very valuable since a considerable proportion of affected infants are stillborn and about half of these deaths occur after the 36th week of pregnancy. Attempts at prediction take into account the amount of anti-D in the mother's plasma, the previous history of affected infants and examination of the bilirubin concentration in the amniotic fluid. None of these are reliable guides when taken singly, but prediction is improved when all three are considered together. Although there are many exceptions, on the whole there is a higher incidence of severe disease in children born to mothers who have high titres of anti-D (values over 256). As mentioned earlier, severe disease tends to run in families and a mother with one stillborn child has approximately a 70% chance of having a second stillbirth. Finally, estimation of the amount of bilirubin spectroscopically in the amniotic fluid at 28 weeks gives some, but by no means a reliable, indication of severity (Fairweather & Walker 1965) and indicates whether premature induction of labour should be carried out at a later date. Since about half the total number of stillbirths occur after the 36th week of pregnancy, induction at 36 weeks reduces the incidence of stillbirth, but this is counterbalanced by the increase in mortality from prematurity.

As soon as the baby is born, cord blood must be obtained and the presence of antibody on the baby's red cells confirmed by the antiglobulin test (p. 134). If this is positive (the strength of the reaction is no guide to severity) then haemoglobulin and plasma bilirubin concentration are estimated, using cord blood. It should be stressed that cord blood is of far greater value than either venous blood or skin prick blood from the child, since the latter normally shows a rise in haemoglobin concentration from about 30 min after birth, due to transfer of blood from the placenta to baby before the cord is tied, followed by a subsequent fall in plasma volume. If the haemoglobin concentration is below the lower limit of normal of 13·5 g/dl an exchange transfusion with Rh-negative blood is required. If the haemoglobin concentration is within the normal range, the decision to give an immediate exchange transfusion rests on the bilirubin concentration. Some pediatricians perform an exchange transfusion if this is above 70 μmoles/l but others have different criteria. Even if the cord haemoglobin concentration is normal, death can still occur from kernicterus if the ability to excrete bilirubin is poorly developed. About half the patients with haemoglobin concentrations within the normal range require an exchange transfusion because of a high bilirubin concentration. The aims of exchange-transfusion are thus twofold.

1   To replace the Rh-positive blood of the child with Rh-negative blood which does not react with anti-D and will thus survive normally. In those relatively rare cases where the antibody concerned is anti-c or anti-E, then blood lacking these antigens is used.

2   To prevent the bilirubin concentration rising to a value of 350 μmoles/l, since kernicterus usually develops if this level is exceeded. Frequent estimations of bilirubin concentration are therefore necessary and several exchange-transfusions may be required.

Prevention of Rh immunization

It is now possible to bring about a very considerable reduction in the incidence of Rh immunization by the injection of anti-D into an Rh-negative mother within 36 hours of giving birth to an Rh-positive child. The injected anti-D combines with the fetal red cells in the mother's circulation and brings about their destruction in the spleen. The precise mechanism by which the suppression of immunization is brought about is not known, but it is assumed that splenic destruction of fetal red cells must divert D antigen on the surface of the cells away from those sites in the immunological system where active antibody production is initiated.

Two observations led to the use of anti-D in the prevention of Rh immunization. First, it was known that anti-D only occasionally developed in the mother if the baby was group A and the mother group O. The suggested explanation of this phenomenon was that the maternal anti-A reacted with the group A fetal red cells and led to their immediate destruction, thus preventing the cells from immunizing the mothers. It was thought that if anti-A could reduce the incidence of immunization, then anti-D might have the same effect. Trials with male volunteers given Rh-positive cells and with women with more than 0·1 ml of fetal cells in their circulation showed that the administration of anti-D would suppress active anti-D production (for reviews, see Clarke 1967 and 1968). Secondly, there was an early immunological observation made by Smith in 1909 and since confirmed many times, that if an antigen is mixed with its specific antibody and injected into an animal, the active antibody response of that animal to the antigen is considerably reduced compared to that seen when the antigen alone is injected. This led a group in New York (Freda *et al*. 1967) independently to carry out trials with anti-D, which were also successful. The injection of anti-D has been shown not only to prevent the appearance of anti-D in the mother 6 months after labour, but also to prevent its appearance during the subsequent pregnancy with an Rh-positive child.

The effectiveness of the treatment will depend partly on the dose of anti-D that is injected. Since the anti-D acts by diverting fetal cells away from stimulating the immunological system, it is reasonable to suppose that the larger the dose, the more effective it will be, especially when the transplacental bleed is a large one. The dose of anti-D that is being used at the moment is 100–300 μg, and there is some evidence that this may protect against a transplacental bleed of 5–15 ml of whole blood. However, it is known that this dose is inadequate against a bleed of 50 ml or more (Dudok de Wit *et al*. 1968) and thus larger doses of anti-D must be given when it is known that the transplacental passage of blood is of this order. In order to detect these large transplacental bleeds, it is necessary to estimate the number of fetal cells in the maternal circulation by the acid-elution technique in every instance when an Rh-positive child is born to an Rh-negative mother.

Preventative immunization has now been used for sufficient time to assess its effectiveness. It would appear that the incidence of HDN in the second Rh-positive child born to a mother who had been treated with anti-D is about 0·5–1%. This figure is to be compared to an incidence of about 17% in untreated women. The failures in preventive therapy are mainly due either to the trans-placental passage at labour of large amounts of fetal red cells (25–50 ml or more) which would not be covered by the standard dose of 100–300 μg of anti-D, or they may be due to primary immunization early in the course of the first pregnancy. The fre-quency of immunization occurring in primigravidae can be consid-erably reduced by the injection of anti-D at 28 weeks of preg-nancy. The combination of anti-D given both at 28 weeks and post-partum can be extremely effective, as has been demonstrated in Manitoba, where all women at risk within the state are treated in this way. The protection rate is over 98%, with the result that perinatal deaths due to HDN have been reduced from about 20 per year to about 1 every 6 years (Bowman & Pollock, 1983).

It is also possible to prevent the production of anti-D when a large amount of Rh-positive blood has been inadvertently trans-fused, the dose of anti-D being of the order of 20 μg for each ml of red cells transfused.

References

BOWMAN J. M. & POLLACK J. (1983) Rh immunization in Manitoba: progress in prevention and management. *Can. Med. Assoc. J.*, **129**, 343.

CLARKE C. A. (1967) Prevention of Rh-haemolytic disease. *Brit. med. J.*, **4**, 7.

CLARKE C. A. (1968) Prevention of Rhesus iso-immunization. *Lancet*, **ii**, 1.

DUDOK DE WIT C., BORST-EILERS E., WEERDT CH. M. V. D. & KLOOSTERMAN G. J. (1968) Prevention of Rhesus Immunization. A controlled clinical trial with a comparatively low dose of anti-D immunoglobulin. *Brit. med. J.*, **4**, 477.

FAIRWEATHER D. V. I. & WALKER W. (1965) Current views on the management of rhesus isoimmunization. *Ob. Gyn. Digest.*, **7**, 49.

FREDA V. J., GORMAN J. G., POLLACK W., ROBERTSON J. G., JENNINGS E. A. & SULLIVAN J. F. (1967) Prevention of Rh isoimmunization. *J. Am. Med. Ass.*, **199**, 390.

GIBLETT E. R. (1964) Blood-group antibodies causing haemolytic disease of the newborn. *Clin. Obstet. Gynec.*, **7**, 1044.

LEVINE P., BURNHAM L., KATZIN E. M. & VOGEL P. (1941) The role of isoimmunization in the pathogenesis of erythroblastosis foetalis. *Am. J. Obs-tet. Gynec.*, **42**, 925.

Recommended reading not mentioned in the text

CLARKE C. A. & McCONNELL R. B. (1972) *Prevention of Rh-hemolytic disease.*
   American Lecture Series, Charles C. Thomas, Illinois.
FULTON R. (1959) Haemolytic disease of the newborn. *Brit. Med. Bull.*, **15**, 119.
WALKER W. (1959) The management of haemolytic disease of the newborn as a
   community problem. *Brit. Med. Bull.*, **15**, 123.
WOODROW J. C. (1970) Rh-immunisation and its prevention. Series *Haematologica*,
   Vol. III, **3**, Munksgaard, Copenhagen.

Objectives in learning: haemolytic disease of the newborn (HDN)

1   To know the cause of HDN, the antigens concerned, the mechanism of immunization and the approximate risk to a mother of becoming immunized.

2   To know the principles of antenatal care concerned with predicting both the presence and severity of the disease.

3   To know the clinical features and extent of variation in severity of HDN, and the causes of disability and death.

4   To know the method of assessment of the severity in the infant immediately after birth and the indications for exchange transfusions.

Chapter 9
Haematological Techniques and Normal Values

This chapter deals only with the basic and common haematological investigations which are in everyday use in a routine haematological laboratory.

Estimation of haemoglobin concentration

The estimation of haemoglobin is dependent on its property of absorbing light in the yellow-green region of the visible spectrum. Since oxyhaemoglobin, reduced haemoglobin, methaemoglobin and carboxyhaemoglobin all absorb light to a different extent, the blood is diluted with a cyanide solution which converts all types of haemoglobin into the stable cyanmethaemoglobin compound. A standard cyanmethaemoglobin solution is used to calibrate the photo-electric colorimeter used for measuring the extent of light absorption. Haemoglobin concentration is expressed as grams of haemoglobin/dl of whole blood.

The accuracy of any particular estimate as carried out in a routine laboratory is difficult to assess, but is probably of the order of ± 5%. The chief sources of error are failure to mix the blood adequately before sampling, and inaccurate dilution.

There is no precise haemoglobin concentration which divides 'normal' from 'abnormal'. Everyone has his own 'normal' haemoglobin concentration which varies slightly according to posture, the altitude at which the person is living (an increase of about 1 g/dl for each kilometre above sea level), and even season of the year. Nevertheless, it is necessary to give arbitrary upper and lower limits for the haemoglobin concentration, based on a survey of a random sample of the population. These limits are fixed so that those whose haemoglobin concentrations fall within the limits need not be investigated further, while those who fall outside probably have some disease and require further investigation. Unfortunately, there is no general agreement as to what the lower limit should be. As Pryce (1960) has pointed out, text books of

Table 9.1

	Lower limit (g/dl)	Upper limit (g/dl)
Pregnant women	11·0	—
Non-pregnant women	12·0	16·5
Men	13·0	18·0

haematology give higher values than those in published surveys of haemoglobin concentrations in apparently healthy people. The lower limits given by text-books of haematology are 13·5–14·0 g/dl for men and 11·5–12·0 g/dl for women. The twelve published surveys quoted by Pryce (1960) give a mean and a standard deviation (assuming a Gaussian distribution within the population); on this basis 95% of normal men have a haemoglobin concentration of approximately 12.0 g/dl or more and 95% of women 11·0 g/dl or more. Pryce suggests that the text-book figures are too high, as they are selected on the basis of ideal normals and that the published surveys give a truer picture of the distribution of haemoglobin concentrations amongst normal people. There is also the problem of defining normal haemoglobin concentrations in pregnancy; it is generally accepted that the normal values are lower at this time, mainly due to an increase in plasma volume.

As long as the uncertainties about the normal range are kept in mind, the lower limits that are recommended for practical use are a compromise between the published figures and are shown in Table 9.1. These values for the lower limits of normal have now been adopted by the World Health Organization (1972).

Children between the ages of 2 months and puberty also have haemoglobin concentrations lower than adults. The lowest level is seen at about 1 year of age, when a haemoglobin concentration in a healthy non-iron-deficient child may be as low as 10 g/dl (Sturgeon 1956).

Estimation of red cell indices

The red cell indices which are of importance in diagnosis are the packed cell volume (PCV), mean cell haemoglobin concentration (MCHC), the mean cell haemoglobin (MCH) and the mean cell volume (MCV).

There are two methods of obtaining these indices, either by manual means, or by the use of electronic counters. Indices derived by manual methods are calculated using 3 basic measurements: haemoglobin concentration, PCV and red cell count. The haemoglobin can be measured spectrophotometrically and the PCV determined by centrifugation of whole blood; both these measurements can be made accurately. The weakness of the manual method lies in the estimate of the red-cell count, estimated by visual counting in a Neubauer or similar type of counting chamber. The results obtained are too inaccurate to be used clinically, so that the only index that can be calculated is the MCHC, which is the haemoglobin concentration divided by the PCV.

Electronic counters, such as the Coulter counter, count the number of red cells accurately as a highly diluted solution of the blood passes through a narrow orifice; they also measure directly the volume of each single red cell. With these two measurements and also an estimation of haemoglobin concentration the MCH, MCHC and PCV are readily calculated.

The question of normal values for the red-cell indices is as uncertain as that of the haemoglobin concentration. Although the electronic counters have improved the precision of measurements (i.e. experimental errors have been considerably reduced), the accuracy (i.e. the relation between the observed result and the true value) has not yet been defined. Electronic counters have to be standardized with a blood sample of known indices, but the difficulty arises in the accurate establishment of these indices. This problem is still being investigated. In the meantime, manufacturers of electronic counters are supplying standards and the use of these appear to give values which are acceptable for clinical use. Generally accepted normal ranges are as follows.

PCV. The normal range is 0·4–0·54 for men, 0·35–0·47 for women (40–54% and 35–47% using the old terminology). The PCV does not supply any more information than is given by the haemoglobin concentration, but is useful for checking the accuracy of the latter.

MCV. The normal range is 76–96 fl (femtolitres). Values below the normal range are found in iron deficiency, thalassaemia major and sometimes in the anaemia of chronic diseases.

MCH. The normal range is 27–32 pg (picograms) (weight of haemoglobin in each cell). Values below normal are found in iron deficiency, thalassaemia major and in some cases of anaemia in chronic diseases.

MCHC. The normal range is 32–36 g/dl. Its main use is in the diagnosis of iron deficiency, but it is not a sensitive index since values only fall consistently below normal when the haemoglobin is below 7 g/dl.

As with the haemoglobin value, a lower range for the values of the indices is found in apparently normal children between the ages of about 3–6 months and 15 years. At one time this was thought to be due to a high prevalence of iron deficiency in children, but it is now clear that children with adequate iron stores have microcytic red cells (by adult standards) with a low MCH as an intrinsic feature of erythropoiesis in childhood. Thus, Hows *et al*. (1977) found a normal range for the MCV of 68–88 fl and MCH of 22–30 pg in children aged 1–6 years. There is a gradual rise in the indices from the time of their lowest values at about 3–12 months of age; adult values are obtained at or shortly after puberty.

Reticulocyte count

Reticulocytes are red cells recently delivered from the marrow and contain the remains of the RNA used in haemoglobin synthesis. The reticulocyte count is the best estimate that we have of the rate of production of viable red cells (p. 49). The RNA is demonstrated by adding red cells to a solution of a supra-vital dye, such as brilliant cresyl blue, which precipitates the RNA as granules and filaments (Plate 3). A film is then made on a slide and the proportion of reticulocytes to total red cells estimated. When the rate of red-cell production is normal, the count in adults does not rise above 2%.

It is more accurate to express the reticulocyte count as the absolute concentration per litre since, when expressed as a percentage, the value is dependent on the total red cell mass. For instance, a value of 2% with a haemoglobin concentration of 14 g/dl would appear as 4% if the haemoglobin was only 7 g/dl. The absolute value varies between 25×10^9 and $85 \times 10^9/l$.

White-cell count

The number of white cells is measured by making a suitable dilution of whole blood and counting visually in a counting chamber. The diluting fluid contains acetic acid, which lyses the red cells, and a dye, such as gentian violet, to stain the white cells. This method is now being superseded by electronic counting methods, which are more accurate and much quicker.

In order to determine the relative proportion of polymorphs, lymphocytes, etc., in the peripheral blood, the distribution in 200 cells on a stained film is determined. The method is not very accurate as the distribution on the stained film is not random: polymorphs and monocytes predominate at the margins and tail of the film and lymphocytes in the centre. Fortunately, when significant deviations from normality occur in patients they are always much greater than the error of the differential count.

The upper limit of normal for the total white-cell count is usually taken to be 10×10^9/l of whole blood, a value of 7×10^9/l for the polymorphs, and 3×10^9/l for lymphocytes, although the latter may be higher than this in infants.

Platelet count

The principle of the method is exactly the same as that for white-cell counts; that is, making a suitable dilution, filling a counting chamber and counting with a moderately high power microscope objective. The diluting fluid that has been found to work well in practice is formaldehyde in saline and no staining is necessary. The normal range for the platelet count is $150-400 \times 10^9$/l. Electronic machines are now available which count platelets far quicker and with far greater accuracy.

Examination of a stained blood film

No haematological diagnosis can be made without examination of a blood film. Therefore, a film should be made and examined on every sample of blood sent to the laboratory, except those sent for blood-clotting tests or for transfusion purposes.

A small drop of blood is spread as a film on a slide and stained with a stain containing methylene blue and eosin. There are various recipes used for making the stain and each has slightly different staining properties. The choice of recipe is immaterial, the essential requirement is consistency in the staining technique. The following information can be obtained from these films.

Red cells

Macrocytes (Plate 1)
If one particular microscope with the same set of lenses is used daily, any abnormality in the diameter of the red cells is instantly recognized. Thus, the increase in diameter of a small proportion of the cells in the macrocytic anaemias of B_{12} and folate deficiencies are readily identified.

Microcytes (Plate 1)
These are cells with diameters below the normal range of approximately 6–8 μm. They are characteristic of iron deficiency and thalassaemia, but are occasionally seen in anaemias associated with chronic infections and neoplasms.

Although microcytes and macrocytes were originally characterized by their diameter as determined by the microscope, they are now also characterized by their cell volume, as determined electronically. The value obtained, expressed in femtolitres (normal range 76–96 fl) is the mean (MCV) for the whole population of red cells examined. As red cells are a heterogenous population with a Gaussian distribution of volumes around the mean, an MCV outside the normal range does not indicate that all the red cells are abnormal, only that more than half are either above or below the normal range of volumes.

Hypochromic cells (Plate 1)
Hypochromic cells have a diminished content of haemoglobin. The central area of the cell fails to stain and the haemoglobin is only present around the periphery. When these cells are seen, the most likely diagnosis is iron deficiency. They are also characteristic of thalassaemia (both homozygous and heterozygous) and are occasionally seen in the anaemia of chronic disorders.

Target cells (Plate 1)
This is a good descriptive term for cells in which the haemoglobin is concentrated centrally and peripherally, with a pale area in between. They are an indication that the cell is abnormally thin and they are seen associated with diseases where haemoglobin produc-

tion is deficient or abnormal, as in iron deficiency and in the haemoglobinopathies. In the latter, the finding of target cells may be the initial indication that an abnormal haemoglobin is present. They are also seen in association with liver diseases.

Polychromatic red cells

In the type of staining used for routine dried-blood films, reticulocytes appear as cells larger than normal. They are stained a diffuse blue-red colour and hence are termed polychromatic cells. The substance staining blue is RNA, which does not precipitate as granules as it does when stained by the supravital technique.

Spherocytes (Plate 2)

In many different types of haemolytic anaemia a few red cells lose their disc shape and become spherical. In stained films, they are recognized as deeply-staining cells of smaller diameter than the normal cells. Spherocytes are an essential feature of hereditary spherocytosis and the diagnosis cannot be made without their presence being established.

Howell–Jolly bodies (Plate 2)

These small round bodies are nuclear remnants and are found in the absence of the spleen. It has been suggested that Howell–Jolly bodies are probably present in normal red cells when they leave the marrow. There is evidence that under normal conditions these bodies are removed by the spleen, possibly during their first passage through that organ, and thus after splenectomy or splenic atrophy, they remain within the red cells in the circulation.

Nucleated red cells; normoblasts (Plate 3)

The only nucleated red cell commonly seen in the peripheral blood is the polychromatic normoblast, the last stage in the development of the red cell. The nucleus is round and deeply staining. Haemoglobin is present in the cytoplasm, which therefore stains blue-red. The presence of these cells in the peripheral blood indicates that there is hyperactivity of red-cell production. They are seen in severe haemolytic anaemias, especially haemolytic disease of the newborn, and they are also seen together with immature white cells when secondary carcinomatous deposits have displaced marrow tissue (leucoerythroblastic anaemia).

White cells

Polymorphs (Plate 4)
Polymorphs are the most numerous of the white cells and are characterized by a multilobed nucleus. Under normal conditions not more than 3% of the polymorphs have five or more lobes, but in B_{12} or folate deficiency, many cells with sex to ten lobes are seen (Plate 4).

Lymphocytes (Plate 5)
These are the cells which produce antibody and are also responsible for cell-mediated immunity. Most lymphocytes are small cells, only slightly larger than a red cell, with only a thin rim of cytoplasm surrounding the nucleus. Most of the lymphocytes are T-cells, only about 10% being B-cells.

Eosinophils
These cells resemble polymorphs in size and in having a multilobed nucleus, but differ from them in that they have large deep red eosinophilic cytoplasmic granules. They have been found to contain inhibitors of various physiologically active substances, of which probably the most imporatant is an inactivator of histamine. This activity could be related to the fact that eosinophilia is frequently seen when immune mechanisms have been stimulated, especially those associated with IgE antibody and the release of histamine from mast cells and basophils. Normal eosinophil counts usually fall within the range $0 \cdot 04 – 0 \cdot 5 \times 10^9/l$ and eosinophilia is frequently associated with asthma, hay fever, urticaria (all involving IgE antibody) and drug sensitization. Eosinophilia also results from the presence of parasites (the most common cause on a world basis) and is also seen in about 20% of cases of exfoliative dermatitis and Hodgkin's disease (Wetherley-Mein 1970).

Immature white cells
These are by definition cells of the myeloid and lymphocytic series that are not normally found in peripheral blood. Their most characteristic feature which makes them easy to identify is their large size, their diameter usually being four or more times larger than that of a red cell. In the myeloid series, the earliest stage of development is the myeloblast (Plate 4); in this cell, nucleoli are

present and there is little cytoplasm. In a later stage (myelocytes, Plate 4), the nucleoli disappear, the cytoplasm increases in volume and contains blue-red staining granules. Microscopists have subdivided the transition from primitive stem cell to mature polymorph into further stages, but no diagnostic advantage is gained from such an analysis.

Heinz bodies (Plate 7)

Ingestion of oxidizing chemicals or drugs may cause denaturation of haemoglobin. This may happen either because the dose of the drug is large, and overwhelms the normal mechanisms for maintaining haemoglobin in the reduced state, or because there is a deficiency of glucose-6-phosphate dehydrogenase; the red cell is then especially sensitive to small doses of oxidizing chemical (p. 58). The denatured haemoglobin precipitates within the cells and can be easily stained using the dye methyl violet. Heinz bodies can be produced *in vitro* by the addition of acetylphenylhydrazine and this can be used as a screening test for glucose-6-phosphate dehydrogenase deficiency, as more Heinz bodies appear in the cells of these patients than in normals.

Bone-marrow biopsy

A sample of bone-marrow can be obtained either by suction through a wide-bored needle from the sternum or iliac crest, or by trephine from the iliac crest. A thin film is spread and stained in the same way as for peripheral blood. The information that can be gained from a bone-marrow biopsy is as follows.

Red-cell series

The presence of hyperplasia or hypoplasia can be assessed. This is usually a subjective assessment based on a knowledge of the density of immature red cells in films made from marrow obtained from normal people. Megaloblastic anaemia is diagnosed by the finding of megaloblasts (Plate 3). These cells are characterized by being larger than normal and having a nucleus which has a much finer reticular network than in normal cells.

White-cell series

As with the red-cell series, it is possible to obtain a subjective estimate of the presence of hyperplasia or hypoplasia. In myeloid leukaemia, there is an increase in the total number of white cells, especially those in an early stage of development (myeloblasts), and abnormal forms and mitotic figures are frequently seen. In lymphocytic leukaemia, there is infiltration with numerous cells of the lymphocytic series.

Megakaryocytes (Plate 8)
The presence or absence of these large characteristic cells is important in the diagnosis of the type of thrombocytopenia (see p. 107). In autoimmune thrombocytopenic purpura, the number of megakaryocytes present is increased.

Iron
Iron stores can be seen as golden-brown granules in the reticulo-endothelial cells of an unstained marrow. Alternatively, the iron can be stained blue with potassium ferricyanide. Visualization of iron in the marrow is an accurate method of assessing iron stores, but serum ferritin levels may be almost as reliable (see p. 14).

Infiltration by other cells
Carcinomatous deposits can be identified in marrow biopsy specimens. In myelomatosis, the marrow is infiltrated with plasma cells.

LE cells

Patients with disseminated lupus erythematosus have an antinuclear antibody in their plasma. The nuclei are phagocytosed by other polymorphs and the LE cell is thus a polymorph containing a pale purple-staining phagocytosed nucleus (Plate 7). The phagocytosis takes place *in vitro* during the hour following withdrawal of blood. A stained blood film is made from the buffy coat after centrifuging.

References

Hows J., Hussein S., Hoffbrand A. V. & Wickramasinghe S. N. (1977) Red cell indices and serum ferritin levels in children. *J. clin. Path.*, **30**, 181.

Pryce J. D. (1960) Level of haemoglobin in whole blood and red blood cells, and proposed convention for defining normality. *Lancet*, **ii**, 333.

Sturgeon P. (1956) Studies of iron requirements in infants and children. *Pediatrics*, **17**, 341.

WETHERLEY-MEIN G. (1970) The significance of eosinophilia. *Practitioner*, **204**, 805.
WHO *Nutritional anaemias* (1972) Technical Bulletin No. 503.

SI units

Haematological values are now expressed in SI units and the agreed form some of the units will take is shown in Table 9.2, which also shows the normal range accepted by many people.

Table 9.2. Normal values for adults

	SI units
Haemoglobin	
Males	13·0–18.0 g/dl
Females	12·0–16·5 g/dl
Females (pregnant)	11·0 g/dl (lower limit)
PCV	
Males	0·40–0·54
Females	0·35–0·47
MCV	76–96 fl
MCH	27–32 pg
MCHC	30–35 g/dl
White-cell count	$4–10 \times 10^9$/l
Platelets	$150–400 \times 10^9$/l
Reticulocytes	$25–85 \times 10^9$/l
Serum iron	10–30 μmol/l
Total iron binding capacity	50–72 μmol/l
Serum B_{12}	150–900 ng/l
Red-cell folate	100–450 μg/l
Serum folate	3–20 μg/l

dl = decilitre (100 ml). fl = femtolitre (1×10^{-15} litre). pg = picogram.

For normal values see Dacie J. V. & Lewis S. M. (1975) *Practical Haematology* (5th edn) Churchill Livingstone, Edinburgh.

Index